Body-Subjects and Disordered Minds

International Perspectives in Philosophy and Psychiatry

Series editors: Bill (K.W.M.) Fulford, Katherine Morris, John Z Sadler,
Giovanni Stanghellini

Volumes in the series:

Forthcoming volumes in the series:

Body-Subjects and Disordered Minds

Eric Matthews

Emeritus Professor of Philosophy and
Honorary Research Professor of Medical and
Pyschiatric Ethics, University of Aberdeen, UK

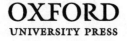

OXFORD
UNIVERSITY PRESS

OXFORD
UNIVERSITY PRESS

Great Clarendon Street, Oxford OX2 6DP

Oxford University Press is a department of the University of Oxford.
It furthers the University's objective of excellence in research, scholarship,
and education by publishing worldwide in

Oxford New York

Athens Auckland Bangkok Bogotá Buenos Aires Cape Town
Chennai Dar es Salaam Delhi Florence Hong Kong Istanbul Karachi
Kolkata Kuala Lumpur Madrid Melbourne Mexico City Mumbai Nairobi
Paris São Paulo Shanghai Singapore Taipei Tokyo Toronto Warsaw

with associated companies in Berlin Ibadan

Oxford is a registered trade mark of Oxford University Press
in the UK and in certain other countries

Published in the United States
by Oxford University Press Inc., New York

© Oxford University Press, 2007

British Library Cataloguing in Publication Data

Data available

Library of Congress Cataloguing in Publication Data

Matthews, Eric, 1936-
Body-subjects and disordered minds / Eric Matthews.
(International perspectives in philosophy and psychiatry)
Includes bibliographical references and index.
ISBN-13: 978-0-19-856644-1 (pbk. : alk. paper)
ISBN-10: 0-19-856644-1 (pbk. : alk. paper)
ISBN-13: 978-0-19-856643-4 (hbk. : alk. paper)
ISBN-10: 0-19-856643-3 (hbk. : alk. paper)
1. Mental illness--Philosophy. 2. Mental illness--Physiological aspects.
3. Psychiatry--Philosophy. 4. Mind and body. I. Title. II. Series.
[DNLM: 1. Mental Disorders--therapy. 2. Mind-Body Relations (Metaphysics)
3. Psychiatry--ethics. WM 400 M438b 2007]
RC437.5.M386 2007
616.89--dc22
2006033357

10 9 8 7 6 5 4 3 2 1

Typeset in Minion
by Cepha Imaging Pvt. Ltd., Bangalore, India.
Printed in Great Britain
on acid-free paper by
Biddles Ltd., King's Lynn, Norfolk

Preface

I have long been puzzled by the notions of 'mental health' and 'mental illness', and have struggled to resolve my bafflement in a number of papers (e.g. Matthews 1995; 2003; 2004; 2005a and forthcoming). At first sight, it might seem strange to be puzzled by these very familiar notions. It seems obvious, after all, that people's thoughts, feelings, desires and behaviour can go wrong, can be 'disordered', just as their hearts, lungs, livers and so on can. When thoughts and so on go wrong, they can create distressing problems for the person concerned: their life is not as good as when things are going right, just as life is not so good when the heart is not going right. When the heart or the liver go wrong, we call in a suitably qualified medical person to try to put things right; and nowadays we are likely also to call on the help of a suitably qualified medical person to deal with at least some of the problems arising when thoughts, feelings, desires and so on awry. In both cases, a 'suitably qualified' medical person is someone who has gone through a standard training in general medicine, and has then specialized in the relevant field. We assume that appropriate medical treatment for thought or mood disorders is of the same general kind as for, say, raised blood pressure or liver problems: medication, nursing care, and, in extreme cases, more radical interventions such as surgery. These treatments do often seem to work, at least in alleviating distress if not in curing the condition.

So where is the puzzle? The answer to that question becomes obvious as soon as one begins to reflect on what has just been said. What is meant by thoughts etc. 'going wrong', and do they go wrong in the same way that hearts and livers do? Talk of thoughts, feelings and desires 'going wrong' seems to imply a reference to some kind of evaluative standard: it may be a cognitive standard, as when someone's thoughts become incoherent or illogical; or a moral standard, as when someone's desires are directed to a disapproved object; or some more general standard of social acceptability, not exactly moral but moral-like, as when someone becomes miserly, or over-anxious, or lacking in self-esteem. None of these ways of going wrong seem to be quite like raised blood pressure or liver failure. The appropriate way to put them right does not seem to be medical or surgical, but something more like education: people with incoherent ideas need to be taught to think more clearly, people with perverse desires to redirect them, people who are over-anxious not to worry so much. Having proper self-esteem, for instance, depends on how one thinks about oneself, on giving due account to one's virtues as well as being critical of one's faults, and it does not seem obvious that taking a pill or having surgery could change one's thoughts in relevant ways. Putting things right seems to be more within one's own control. It becomes easier to see, therefore, why, in popular thinking at least, failure to put things right comes to be seen as open to condemnation or stigma.

Similarly, is the distress caused by things going wrong with one's thoughts, feelings, and desires of the same kind as that caused by things going wrong with one's bodily processes? Headaches, stomach aches, tingling sensations in the extremities, sharp stabbing pains, a general lassitude and debility and the like, are typical results of bodily illness. Some of these may also be found in some forms of mental disorder, but not all: what is more characteristic of mental disorder are such things as feelings of sadness and bewilderment, difficulties in forming relationships, an inability to hold down a job, a refusal of food, feelings of panic. But these are also found in people who are not regarded as mentally ill, and may also be consequences of bodily illness. Where do we draw the line between normal human distress and difficulty in living and that which is the result of mental disorder – or is it a matter of degree? Is there a sharp distinction between mental disorder and bodily illness? And is what we mean by 'mental health' a feeling of contentment, or an ability to manage one's own life, or what? No such difficulties seem to attend the definition of bodily health.

These problems are not just theoretical: they have a bearing on actual clinical practice, which cannot proceed satisfactorily without some thought about key concepts like those of mental health, mental illness, bodily health and illness, the way in which we should explain them and treat them, and so on. They also give rise to special problems in the ethics and law of mental health, in deciding on the responsibility of those who are mentally ill for their actions, and on questions of consent to treatment. To try to solve these practical problems requires, in my view, some philosophical reflection, and that is why I have written this book As a philosopher, who has engaged for the past twenty years or so in fairly constant dialogue with psychiatrists and others in the mental health field, I have become increasingly convinced that the questions will remain unanswered if we do not do some hard philosophical thinking about the concepts used in formulating them. Above all, we need to think rigorously about what is meant by 'mind' and 'mental', and how it relates to what is meant by 'body' and 'bodily'. Traditionally (and especially since the seventeenth century), our culture has been in the grip of two opposed conceptions of the mental, which are nevertheless parasitic on each other. On the one hand, we have thought of the mind as a unique kind of thing, made of different stuff from everything else in the created universe and obeying different laws. This non-material mind is supposed to be found *within* each human individual, discoverable only by that individual, by means of introspection. On the other hand, and more typical of a science-based society, we have thought of the mind as identical with the brain, an ordinary material thing made of the same stuff as everything else in the universe and governed by the same laws as them.

The opposition between these two views, and the arguments for and against each of them, are familiar to anyone with even the slightest acquaintance with modern philosophy. They are also held, as articles of faith, by people who know little or nothing about the philosophical debate: the non-material view mainly by those who think it essential to religious belief, the material view by those who think it is the only one compatible with a truly scientific outlook. I want to argue, however, that both are inadequate as a basis for thinking about mental disorder and its treatment. Instead, I want to present and argue for a third conception – the account given by the French philosopher, Maurice Merleau-Ponty (1908–1961). According to Merleau-Ponty, we should not think of 'minds' and 'bodies', but rather of *human beings*, seen as subjects who are essentially embodied. The thoughts, feelings, desires and so on that we have are not things or processes going on inside us, but ways in which we, as embodied subjects, relate to the world of things, people and cultural objects and institutions: ways in which we are, as he would put it, 'in-the-world'. They explain our behaviour not as causes, governed by general laws, but by providing reasons for doing what we do: since what we do is defined by the concepts which we, along with others in our culture, apply to it. To be in the world in the way in which human beings are is on this view essentially to be *embodied*: we are not just subjects, but 'body-subjects', as it is often expressed. Our subjectivity – our thoughts, feelings, desires, intentions – is necessarily expressed in, and constrained by, the structures of our bodies. Understanding the mind, and so mental disorder, then becomes a matter of understanding the various ways in which our being-in-the-world can be related to the nature of our embodiment, and in particular to our brain processes.

One beneficial consequence of this way of thinking, in my opinion, is that it loosens up our thinking about mental disorder, and the need for such loosening up is the main conclusion of this book. We do not need, I shall argue, to treat all the conditions we call mental disorders in the same way, because 'mind' is not the name of any unified thing, but a way of referring to a set of human attributes and capacities, loosely related in that they are all intentional – a term which will be explained in the course of the book. We do not need, therefore, to be stuck with simple dichotomies – is the medical model applicable to mental disorder, or is it not? Is mental disorder an illness or is it not? Perhaps it is helpful to think in medicalized terms about some aspects of some mental disorders, but not so helpful about other aspects, and maybe what is meant by 'thinking in medicalized terms' may vary from context to context. Some mental disorders may be illnesses and others not; and even those which are may have important differences from bodily illnesses. Another dichotomy which I shall question is that between the conception of mental illness as caused by brain disease and as understandable as a human response to terrible situations. This distinction is founded, I shall argue, in a confused account of the nature of explanation. Similarly, the question whether mentally ill offenders are 'mad or bad' is, I shall conclude, posed in far too simple terms: deciding whether mental illness excuses may be, and I shall argue is, a matter for complex and subtle thought about the varieties of mental disorder. In short, it is not the aim of this book to offer clear-cut answers to such over-simplified questions, but to make clear just how over-simplified the questions are. I approach the area with trepidation, since I am a philosopher with no clinical experience: some of the examples I give in illustration may indeed seem to practitioners to be lacking in clinical reality. That need not matter if they make the essential point clear: it is always open to readers to find better examples.

This book has benefited from the input of more people than I can remember or mention. As I said earlier, I have been discussing these issues over many years, in the context of the Royal College of Psychiatrists Philosophy Special Interest Group, and more recently at meetings of the International Network for Philosophy of Psychiatry, and have gained much from the comments and criticisms of psychiatric and philosophical colleagues at these meetings. Still, if I am to single out particular individuals, I must mention a number of people who have been particularly influential and whom I feel privileged to count as friends: Bill Fulford (above all), Grant Gillett, Gerrit Glas, Giovanni Stanghellini, John Sadler, Jennifer Radden, Julian Hughes, Man Chung, Alan Wear, Iain McGilchrist, John Callender, David Findlay and Martin Wylie. To all of these I am profoundly grateful, as I am to my wife Hellen for her patience with my preoccupations and the insights which she has contributed from her own experience.

Aberdeen   Eric Matthews
June 2006

Contents

Chapter 1

Introducing the problem

Mental disorder

A culture can be regarded, from one point of view, as constituted by sets of rules. Some of these rules will be moral in character: respect other people's property, tell the truth, don't kill, help those in distress, and so on. Some moral rules will have the sanction of law, as in the case of the laws against murder and theft. Some will not: but the moral rules will express the values of the culture in question, its ideas about what a good life is like. Other sorts of rules will be rules of aesthetics, or of etiquette. But there is one kind of rule which is particularly relevant to the subject matter of this book. These are rules of what can be called, in a rather vague sense, 'rationality' – rules determining what counts as rational and what does not. Included in this category will certainly be the rules of logic: it is not rational to believe in two mutually contradictory propositions at the same time – for instance, that someone is both dead and alive.

However, rationality is not a matter only of logicality. Beliefs can be held to be irrational even if they are not self-contradictory – as when someone believes something in the face of a mass of obviously contrary evidence – and rationality or its opposite can also be a feature of behaviour, emotions, wishes, desires and even hopes, to which logic in the strict sense does not apply. It is not rational, for instance, knowingly to act against one's own long-term self-interest, or to pursue minimal benefit at great risk or great cost. It is not rational to feel emotions which are inappropriate to, or disproportionate to, their objects. It is not rational to wish for the moon, or to desire to be a famous film star if one has neither good looks nor acting ability nor any contact with film studios. Nor is it rational to fail to control one's behaviour when it is socially inappropriate, for example, to fail to control one's sexual desires, or desire to utter obscenities, in situations where such behaviour would give offence.

There is a sense in which standards of rationality can vary from culture to culture. It is always irrational to believe two mutually contradictory propositions at the same time, but cultures may differ in what they regard as contradictory. To non-believers, or believers in other religions, for example, it might seem that believing in a God who is both one person and three is believing something contradictory; but to Christians, belief in a triune God is simply orthodoxy, and any appearance of contradiction is merely due to the limitations of our understanding. Similarly, what counts as adequate evidence for a belief may vary from culture to culture: belief in witches, for example, probably seemed like simple common sense to people in the Middle Ages, whereas it appears entirely irrational to a scientifically minded person in twenty-first century Europe. The risk–benefit calculation can also vary: a Homeric hero was expected to be willing to take much greater risks for what might seem to us to be small benefits than, say, a modern accountant. And what counts as proportionate or appropriate emotion can vary from one culture to another: to marry only for love may seem completely reasonable behaviour in modern Western culture, but utterly foolish in a society in which marriages are arranged by families. Likewise, to swear compulsively might be seen as totally inappropriate when walking along a city street, but perfectly normal in a group of soldiers. 'Rational', in this vague sense, seems to mean much the same as 'intelligible to most people', and what is intelligible behaviour or an intelligible thought or emotion in one context, or to one group of people, may not be so in another place or to other people.

All human beings behave irrationally to some extent. Even the attempt to be 'perfectly rational' – for instance, to organize one's life scientifically – can, paradoxically, be seen as a form of irrationality: a sensible person allows room for emotion and imagination as well as rationality in this sense. Most of us harbour beliefs based on very little evidence, or are prepared in some circumstances to take quite unjustifiable risks, or wish for impossible things, or fall in love with rather unsuitable people. In some cases, however, irrationality of thought, behaviour, emotion, wish, desire, and so on exceeds all normal limits, either in its extent or in the length of time it lasts: so much so that it makes someone's life with others almost impossible, or leads to actions which are morally or legally unacceptable, such as random attacks on innocent people. Breaches of the standards of rationality of a society can, in the latter cases, overlap with breaches of its moral norms. When irrationality does exceed its 'normal' bounds in these ways, we are inclined to call it mental disorder, or even, in its most extreme forms, madness. But of course the bounds of normality are liable to be as culturally variable as concepts of irrationality in general. What one culture thinks of as a religious maniac may in another be seen as a person of exceptional (and admirable) piety. What one society regards as a dashing Casanova may be thought of in another as a man with disturbed sexuality.

Is mental disorder an illness?

Whatever variations there may be in the kinds of behaviour, thought, emotion and so on which are included in the class of mental disorders, all societies have to recognize that some of their members will be disturbed in mind in this sense. All cultures have therefore to take account of the concept of mental disorder, both intellectually, in their thinking about such people, and practically, in their dealings with them in morality, law and other institutions. Intellectually, this is a matter of making sense of the way in which human beings can differ so radically from the norm. Different cultures handle the concept in different ways. Some will assimilate mental disorder to moral disorder: mentally disordered people, on this view, are morally depraved, or vicious, or perverted, or degenerate. They have allowed themselves to degenerate from the human level and conduct themselves like the beasts of the field. There is a remnant of this way of thinking in the modern popular usage of the term 'sick' in relation to minds: those who are described as having 'sick minds' are mainly those who are sexually deviant, such as paedophiles, or rapists, or avid consumers of pornography. The use of the word sick in this context does not carry any implications that the sick person deserves compassion (as it does when we say that someone is sick with cancer): rather it is a term of criticism – a 'sick' person is someone to be condemned, and even more strongly than someone who merely does wrong in what we consider to be a more 'normal', human way. The stigma which often attaches to mental disorder, even now, is to some extent a result of this way of thinking: to have a mental disorder is to be different from normal people, in a sense which implies that one falls below the acceptable level of conduct, thought or emotion, of the rest of society. (The stigma can also arise from assimilating mental disorder to mental disability, to falling below the normal *intellectual* level). Plato, who is cited by Anthony Kenny (Kenny 1969) as the inventor of the term 'mental illness', in fact goes on to reject medical treatment for this kind of illness in favour of punishment by judges, thus showing that he understood 'illness' in the same way as modern popular usage understands 'sickness'. But of course mental disorder can be plausibly identified with moral disorder only in those cases where it is expressed in behaviour of kinds which would normally be thought of as morally wrong. Phobias, for example – irrational fears of open spaces, or heights, or spiders – are certainly cases of mental disorder but can hardly be regarded as worthy of moral condemnation.

Other cultures have thought of mental disorder as the result of possession by spirits. Those who suffer from mental disorder are said to have lost their humanity, or reason, and been taken over by non-human (probably subhuman) spirits who now direct their activities. The possessed are not to be condemned for being as they are, but they are to be shunned as dangerous and uncontrollable, immune to any ordinary rational means of persuasion. If they are to be treated, it must be by some method which will drive out the evil spirits from them and allow their humanity to return. Most of the methods for driving out the spirits are fairly harsh and punitive. Again, this interpretation of mental disorder only plausibly applies to certain kinds of disordered behaviour which look scarcely human: for instance, that which deviates from normal decency, or perhaps is abnormally flamboyant in character, in the way in which madness is traditionally conceived. This association of mental disorder with possession by alien forces is, again, partly responsible for the stigma which often attaches to those with such problems.

Both these views of mental disorder have featured in the history of Western culture, and elements of them still persist, at least in popular thinking. The view which has come to be dominant, at least officially, in modern Western society is that of mental disorder as mental *illness*. Mental illness, on this conception, is seen as parallel to bodily illness, as the latter is conceived in modern scientific medicine. This 'medical model' of mental disorder, as it is often called, is understandably regarded as the only possible way for an enlightened person in a scientific culture to think of the bizarre, unintelligible, ways of thinking, acting, feeling, desiring and so on to which some of our fellow human beings are subject. They are not, on this view, to be condemned or shunned for being like this, any more than someone is to be condemned or shunned for having cancer or measles. (Someone with an infectious disease like measles might be isolated temporarily to prevent the risk of spreading the disease, but that is not the same as shutting them away in permanent isolation from normal society, or in harsh conditions). They should not be stigmatized, but treated with sympathy, like other sufferers. Indeed, it is important on this view to see them as *suffering* from mental illness and its consequences, as *patients*, in the same way that those with bodily illnesses suffer from their conditions and their consequences. The aim, in both cases, should be to cure the illness, or at least to alleviate its symptoms, so that the sufferer can be restored to health and to living, as other healthy people do, in normal society. Even when mental illness is expressed in acts which would otherwise be criminal, the sufferers should be sympathized with as such: not punished, but treated, to relieve their suffering as well as to save society at large from some of its consequences.

On the medical model, psychiatry becomes a branch of medicine, alongside such specialties as urology or cardiology. Psychiatrists should therefore have a general medical training before they specialize in their particular field.

They work in hospitals or clinics, or in private practice. They offer diagnoses like other medical practitioners, fitting their patients' conditions into established diagnostic categories – schizophrenia, depression, agoraphobia, personality disorder, dementia, and the like. These diagnoses are at present based mainly on outwardly observable symptoms – behavioural traits, peculiar affects or desires, ways of talking or thinking etc., but the hope is, as in general medicine, that it will be possible eventually, with sufficient research, to identify the causes in the malfunctioning of particular organs which give rise to these symptoms, and to base diagnosis on these causes rather than the symptoms. One organ above all is seen as the most likely place to look for these causes, namely, the brain. After all, thought, feeling, intention to act, desire, and so on all clearly involve the brain, and the greater our knowledge of the brain and how it works, the more we seem to understand about the connections between brain function and chemistry and those features of human beings we think of as belonging to their mental life. So the treatments which are offered for mental illness, on the medical model, are those which are thought likely to affect the brain – drugs to influence brain chemistry, or in some cases surgery to correct defects in brain functioning, or treatments like electroconvulsive therapy to affect electrical activity in the brain.

The medical model has had undeniable success in many ways. Treating mental disorder medically, by means of drugs and occasionally surgery and other physical therapies has helped many, many people to live lives which are more like those which most of us are able to lead, and which they themselves find more satisfactory. They may not be perfectly happy, but then neither are most 'normal' people: and ordinary unhappiness, as I understand Freud once said, is preferable to neurotic misery. No one who has seen the transformation sometimes produced by medication in the lives of those suffering from schizophrenia or serious depression can doubt the value of these treatments. This in itself lends force to the idea that mental disorder is an illness, requiring medical treatment – in other words, to the medical model.

Anti-psychiatry

Alongside what we may call the official view of mental disorder in modern culture, however, there is a persistent current of opposition to the medical model. This movement is often called 'anti-psychiatry', though not all of those opposed to the medical model would accept that label, and their views are very diverse in character, united more by what they oppose than by the way in which they oppose it. Anti-psychiatry has been much discussed and analysed, and it would be tediously and superfluously repetitious to go over that discussion again here, except in so far as it is relevant to advancing the themes of this book. It will be sufficient to say that some writers are given this label because they oppose drug treatments as being allegedly too much dominated by big international drug companies, interested in profit rather than human welfare. Furthermore, many would claim that drug treatments are liable to have undesirable side-effects which outweigh any benefits which they may bring, and are anyway more a matter of controlling the behaviour of patients to make them easier to manage than of relieving the patients' suffering. Others oppose the medical model on more philosophical grounds. Thomas Szasz (as in Szasz 1972) regards the whole notion of mental illness as a myth, enabling social deviants to be controlled by doctors under the guise of treatment, and so denied any real human dignity for their choice of lifestyle. A variant of this is Foucault's conception of scientific psychiatry as an example of the way in which, in modern culture, power is exercised by the use of scientific methods to manipulate deviants into willing acceptance of their own subordination (see Foucault 1989). In the case of R. D. Laing (see Laing 1965), a medicalized conception is rejected because it denies the possibility of seeing what we call mental disorder as an experience which may give greater insight into reality than that of those people we call normal.

The first version of anti-psychiatry is essentially political. It is not really incompatible with a view of mental disorder as illness, but rather a criticism of the methods currently used to treat the illness. This criticism, moreover, is concerned with the power relations between pharmaceutical companies and the mentally ill and their carers, or between doctors and their patients, rather than going to the heart of the concept of mental illness itself. Its validity depends to a large extent on empirical facts about the characteristics of current drug treatments and prescribing practices, rather than on any conceptual analysis. For these reasons, it is not really appropriately discussed in a philosophical work such as this. The other versions of anti-psychiatry mentioned – those of Szasz, Foucault and Laing – are more clearly philosophical in character, and so I shall concentrate on them.

In their different ways, anti-psychiatrists of this second sort question the whole conception of mental disorder as an illness, comparable to bodily illnesses such as cancer or measles. Being mentally disordered is seen by them not as suffering from a condition caused by external factors, but rather as being socially deviant, in the sense of behaving and thinking in ways which transgress the ordinary norms of social life. Some, such as Szasz, seem to regard the term illness as only literally applicable to bodily conditions (Szasz 1972: 10). If so, then the expression 'mental illness' is either an oxymoron, or at best a rather misleading metaphorical extension of the meaning of illness.

Moreover, for Szasz, it seems that what is mental is what is freely chosen, so that a mental disorder must be a form of behaviour which the person in question has deliberately adopted. It is a strategy for dealing with the problems which face one. The adoption of this strategy may certainly cause problems for the person in question: it may be an *inappropriate* or *ineffective* way of dealing with his or her situation. It then becomes what Szasz calls a 'problem in living', by which he seems to mean the sort of problem which the normal free agent encounters in the course of living – such as a difficulty in a personal relationship, or in coping with the demands of a job, or in managing one's finances. Problems of this kind are clearly not such as to require medical treatment in any ordinary sense: sound advice from someone sympathetic is most likely to help.

Foucault, on the other hand, sees those who are described as mad as people whom conventional bourgeois society finds difficulty in fitting in to its framework, and consequently needs to control. The idea of mental disorder as illness simply reflects, in his view, the way in which we seek in modern society to control such deviants, not by the exercise of naked force, but by labelling them as sick and in need of medical treatment. It is a way in which those with power in society disguise their own domination over others. Laing, on the other hand (who, it is important to note, rejected the 'anti-psychiatry' label, but has important elements of similarity with the anti-psychiatrists), was much more aware than either Szasz or Foucault of the depth of the problems faced by those described as mentally ill, in particular by patients with schizophrenia, who were his main concern. But he saw this suffering not as the result of an illness – something wrong within the sick person – but as the outcome of his or her problems in dealing with the contradictions of conventional society. The expressions of schizophrenia – apparently meaningless babbling, thought insertion, and the like – were not symptoms of an illness, like the spots which indicate measles, but an attempt to communicate the schizophrenic's bafflement in the face of the confusing responses of others to him or her (Laing 1965: 29ff.). As such they could, perhaps with great difficulty and the exercise of imagination, be *understood*, in the same way as any other human expression. At worst, they could be seen as like someone speaking a foreign language, which must be learned before it can be understood; or like someone expressing very new and original ideas which are hard for ordinary, relatively unoriginal people to grasp. Laing does indeed speak on occasion about the way in which the 'cracked' mind of the schizophrenic can let in more light than the solid mind of the 'normal' person (Laing 1965: 27).

The main problem with all of these more philosophical forms of rejection of the medical model is that, in rejecting the idea of mental disorder as an illness, they also in effect deny the very real suffering which mentally disordered people can experience. Treating mental disorder as the adoption of an inadequate strategy for coping with problems in living seems to devalue this suffering: a strategy for coping is something we choose to adopt, not something which a cruel fate causes us to suffer. This conception seems particularly misguided, and even inhuman, in regard to such conditions as schizophrenia or depression. Foucault's depiction of mad people as effectively rebels against the established order diminishes the suffering which these conditions entail even more obviously. A rebel may be admirable, but is not, like the victim of involuntary pain or distress, the object of sympathy. Laing, as we saw earlier, does have more of a sense of the suffering of schizophrenics and other mentally disordered people than Szasz or Foucault, and is in this way more humane in his attitudes towards mental disorder than them. Nevertheless, his tendency to romanticize schizophrenics as prophets and seers conflicts with this sense of schizophrenia as a source of real suffering. Great original thinkers do suffer from being out of tune with the stuffy, conventional world around them, but the suffering is perhaps more bearable because it can be offset against the feeling that one has something new to communicate: it is the necessary price to pay for being as one is, and being as one is is a good thing. The schizophrenic's suffering is not made bearable in this way: it is not so much like the sense of being special that the original thinker may experience, but more like the isolation and alienation of someone who does not fit in with others yet longs to do so. Even the ability to manage schizophrenia, or depression, or other mental disorders, acquired by the use of medication, is experienced as a liberation, not a restriction. Life may be duller, but it is at least more bearable. (For further critical discussion of Laing and Szasz, see Matthews [2005] and Matthews [forthcoming]).

Anti-psychiatry, then, while it may suggest new and useful ways of thinking about mental disorder (and I shall later argue for some of these ways of thinking), ultimately misses something important about these forms of human misery which is properly caught by the word illness. It fails to identify what the real problem is in the concept of mental illness. Still, as I shall argue in the next section, there are reasons other than those of the anti-psychiatrists for finding difficulty in the medical model as presently understood. If we can examine those, they may help us to identify the nature of the problem (or problems) more accurately, and in a way which suggests more promising ways of resolving the problem.

Problems in the medical model

Even if we do not accept the arguments of such thinkers as Szasz, Laing and Foucault, there are good reasons for discontent with at least the present understanding of the medical model of mental disorder. There are features, even within our current ways of dealing with mental disorder, which do not fit well with the medical model as stated so far, crucial to which is a certain conception of what *medicine* is. The medical model so conceived sees psychiatry as a branch of *scientific* medicine, which, like other branches, requires a preliminary training in knowledge of the human body and how it works and may fail to work. Medicine is scientific, in that it diagnoses and treats illness as an expression of malfunction (disease) in some bodily organ or system. Diagnosis and treatment thus require knowledge of the proper functioning of bodily organs or systems, of how that can go wrong, and of how it can be treated to correct that malfunction and restore health. No treatment can be scientific unless it is based on evidence of an actual effect on functioning produced by it. This implies that scientific treatments must be physical, in the sense of the administration of some substance which is known to have such an effect, in accordance with established scientific laws; or else of some kind of surgical intervention which will again have a known effect on the way in which the bodily process in question proceeds.

If we look around us at the actual treatments we offer to people with mental disorders, however, we see that this picture is not entirely accurate. Many of those who treat mental problems, for one thing, have no medical training – which is not to say that they are *un*trained, still less that they are quacks, but that they have other kinds of training – in psychology or social work, for example, and the treatments which they offer are not of the standard medical kind: they are what are described as 'talking therapies' – treatments which consist in the therapist talking to the patient (more likely called the client in a further divergence from the medical model), with a view to changing the client's own perception of their condition. Even medically trained psychiatrists may well offer such talking cures, perhaps in addition to medication, but no one, except a quack, would suggest treating cancer or measles by talking to the patient about his or her perceptions of what was wrong.

It might be (and probably would be) suggested by defenders of this version of the medical model that we should not pay too much attention to the practice of psychotherapy or talking treatments. The existence of such practices, they might say, tells us nothing about the real nature of mental illness, but only about the present unsatisfactory state of psychiatry. It is in a relatively primitive or undeveloped condition, they might say, and has not yet become fully scientific. Above all, the talking therapy implies a belief in the independent causal influence of such things as thoughts, emotions, wishes, intentions – in short of 'mental' entities – but this, they would argue, is contrary to what is required by a genuinely scientific philosophy. Thoughts and intentions must, in such a philosophy, be identified with brain processes, which are publicly observable and measurable, and whose causal influence can be studied in other cases. Or else, still more radical, we should, as those philosophers called eliminative materialists argue, regard all this talk of thoughts and motives as simply part of a primitive, pre-scientific, theory of human behaviour (folk-psychology, to use their derogatory term), which ought simply to be eliminated in favour of a developed neuroscience. In a properly scientific psychiatry, the talk would only be of neurons and neurotransmitters, both in the explanation of disordered behaviour and, consequently, in its treatment. (There will be a fuller discussion of eliminative materialism in a later chapter). On this view, psychotherapy is a pre-scientific, essentially magical, mode of treatment: psychotherapists are, as it were, a kind of witch doctor.

It is easy to see why this line of thought seems appealing, but it does not have as much force as its proponents believe. Too much is taken for granted which is in fact open to question. A scientific approach, to begin with, surely cannot be equated with a particular metaphysics, such as the brain–mind identity theory or eliminative materialism. To be scientific is to seek for the most empirically adequate account of the phenomena, rather than the one which best conforms to some favoured philosophical account of them. Philosophy ought to follow science, rather than the other way around. There are grounds for thinking that concepts like thought, belief, wish, motive, and so on cannot be eliminated from any explanation of human behaviour which would be adequate to the phenomena. For example, both a highly competitive businessman and a violent criminal exhibit aggressive tendencies: if we are to explain the difference between the ways in which they express their aggression, can we do so without invoking their own *thoughts* about their aims? The businessman's aggression is channelled into commercial competition, the criminal's into, say, mugging old ladies and stealing their purses. The difference does not seem to be explicable without some reference to the concepts of commercial competition and mugging, and to the understanding of these concepts by the two men. (This argument will be developed more fully later in the book.)

It is at least questionable, then, whether the practice of psychotherapy is merely a sign of scientific underdevelopment in psychiatry. If it is not, then we may also question whether a scientific conception of mental disorder is necessarily one which conceives of and treats it as brain disease. We might also be led to ask whether this affects our conception of illness, and so of the medical model, in general. Perhaps what needs to be examined is not so much whether mental disorder is an illness, but whether we are trying to operate with an inadequate conception of illness (which may even have relevance to the case of bodily illness). Putting it differently, maybe it is not so much a matter of deciding whether the medical model applies to mental disorder, as of revising our view of what the medical model entails, to make it fit mental disorder.

Diagnosis

This has a bearing on another difficulty with the medical model as currently interpreted. A scientific medicine is supposed to be one based on objective disease classifications. Patients present to doctors with certain symptoms – they have headaches, or skin rashes, or difficulty in urinating, and so on. These symptoms may seem to cluster in groups, and an initial formulation of a disease concept may be based on such a cluster. The cluster may, of course, only be apparent: what looks like different symptoms of the same disease may, in fact, be symptoms of more than one associated disease. This is important in choosing the best treatment. A disease classification based only on appearances of clustering is subjective in an obvious sense. An objective classification would be one based on real clusters, and that must surely mean clusters which are grouped together because they are all the effects of a common cause. The cause, in the case of bodily illness at least, is generally taken to be some problem with an internal organ: the symptoms are external signs that something is wrong with the heart, or kidneys, or genito-urinary system, or the lungs, or whatever.

It is this 'something wrong inside' which a scientific medicine seeks to treat. Diagnosis is the business of identifying what is wrong inside, on the basis of the external symptoms (together of course with such things as the patient's medical history, recent exposure to potential causes of things going wrong in these ways, and so on). All of this is entirely objective: what is a symptom of what, and what counts as going wrong, are supposed to be matters of fact, independent of what the patient or the doctor thinks, or of any value judgements which may be made in one culture rather than another. According to the conceptions of scientific medicine as currently understood, for instance, whether or not a certain kind of seizure is a symptom of epilepsy is independent of how anyone experiences or thinks about such seizures; and whether or not epilepsy is a disease, and distinct from other diseases with similar symptoms, is independent of the way in which seizures are evaluated in particular value systems.

A psychiatry modelled on scientific medicine ought to follow the same pattern. There ought to be objectively distinguished mental disorders, which psychiatrists ought to diagnose on the basis of recognized symptoms and then treat appropriately. Moreover, these recognized clusters of symptoms ought to have their basis in a common cause, located in the patient's body. 'Official' psychiatry does indeed attempt to follow this model. Diagnostic classifications have been devised to provide the basis for proper psychiatric diagnoses, by listing the distinctive signs of particular conditions: those most used at present are the World Health Organization's (1992) ICD-10 (*International Classification of Diseases*, tenth revision) and the American Psychiatric Association's (1994) DSM-IV (*Diagnostic and Statistical Manual of Mental Disorders*, fourth Edition). Unfortunately, the actuality does not entirely correspond to the ideal represented by these classifications. Even some of those involved in producing them would admit that it is difficult even to formulate a satisfactory concept of a mental disorder. For example, Professor Allen J. Frances MD, the Chair of the DSM-IV Task Force, says,

> DSM-IV is a manual of *mental disorders*, but it is by no means clear just what *is* a mental disorder and whether one can develop a set of definitional criteria to guide inclusionary and exclusionary decisions for the manual.
>
> (in Sadler, Wiggins and Schwartz 1994: vii)

There are disputes, for instance, about whether alcoholism is a mental illness or not, or autism, or antisocial behaviour, or ADHD (the nature of the dispute differs from case to case). There have been heated arguments about whether homosexuality is a mental disorder, though most would now agree that it is not. There are questions about whether certain alleged mental disorders actually exist or not: for instance, psychopathy or dissociative identity disorder (formerly called multiple personality disorder). There are questions about whether, say, schizophrenia is one disorder or many, and at the level of clinical practice, it is often difficult to decide whether a patient is suffering from schizophrenia or severe depression.

It may well be said, and with justification, that it is also true in general medicine that diagnosis presents problems which at least appear similar. Is 'post-viral syndrome' a genuine illness? Is there such a thing as 'Gulf War syndrome'? Is cancer one disease or many? In clinical practice, diagnosis is often problematic in the case of bodily as well as mental disorders, but there are significant differences. When we ask whether what looks like a bodily illness is really a medical condition or not, we very often mean, is it really organic or merely psychosomatic? The issue, in other words, is whether the condition is 'only in the mind' – hardly a question it makes sense to ask about alleged mental disorders. Second, we can always hope, with alleged bodily conditions, to settle the matter in a reasonably objective way, by investigating bodily organs and systems: and the history of medicine would support that hope. Whether or not post-viral syndrome is more than merely imaginary or in the mind could in principle be established beyond doubt by thorough examination of sufferers' bodies. Similarly, the practical clinical problems can in principle be resolved by internal examination. In the case of psychiatric diagnosis, on the other hand, this method of definitive settlement of the questions does not seem to be available, at least at present. Both DSM-IV and ICD-10 for the most part classify conditions by symptoms or diagnostic signs alone, not by the internal causes of these external signs: for example, ICD-10 characterizes the schizophrenic disorders by 'fundamental and characteristic distortions of thinking and perception, and by inappropriate or blunted affect' (World Health Organization 1992: 86). This is no accident, since we are far from knowing at present whether most mental disorders even have internal or organic causes, still less what those causes might be.

Once again, a defender of the medical model, as so far presented, might object that this is simply an outcome of the scientifically undeveloped nature of psychiatry at present, not an indication of anything essential or fundamental about mental disorder. 'You say', the defender might respond, 'that we don't know *at present* whether schizophrenia has organic causes, or if so what they might be: but it doesn't follow that we shall never know. There have been many cases in the history of medicine in which causes which were unknown at one time have later been discovered: surely, we have every reason to hope that psychiatric diagnosis will one day be put on a proper scientific basis in the same way. All that is needed is more research, in particular in genetics or neuroscience or both.'

But does the parallel really hold? There seem to be conceptual difficulties in the assumption that the development of psychiatric explanation will necessarily follow that of explanation in general medicine. The symptoms of bodily illness are themselves bodily states and processes – fatigue, physical pain, rashes, high temperatures, and the like. It is reasonable to suppose, therefore, that they have similarly bodily causes, which, if we do not already know them, can be established by appropriate research. The symptoms of mental disorder are such things as thoughts, feelings, beliefs, moods, ways of perceiving, and these are not physical states, unless one accepts a brain–mind identity thesis or eliminative materialism (which, it was argued earlier, cannot be simply assumed to be true). It is far from obvious, therefore, that they can be completely explained by bodily processes.

Indeed, it could be argued that they certainly can *not* be completely explained in this way. Take, for instance, the delusive belief that the man over there is an agent of an international conspiracy which is out to get me. This belief has two features which, at least prima facie, distinguish it from a bodily event or state. First, it is subjective, in the sense that it exists only as held by some subject; second, it is intentional: it is essentially directed towards the outside world. (This is Brentano's sense of the word intentional, which will be discussed further in Chapter 5, not the standard sense in which it means roughly the same as deliberate). The same could be said about other typical symptoms of mental disorder, such as emotions. An emotion such as anxiety, for instance, is necessarily *someone's* emotion, and it is anxiety *about* something. This makes them different from the typical symptoms of bodily disease, in a number of ways, in particular in the way they can be explained. We can explain the delusive thought mentioned above, for example, only if we can explain the norms of rationality in terms of which it is delusive. Because of the subjectivity and intentionality of belief, someone can only be said to hold the belief that someone else is intent on killing him if he knows what that proposition means, that is, what fact would make it true. That implies also that someone must have grounds for believing – reasons for thinking that it is true in the relevant circumstances – which he himself regards as adequate. Calling the belief in this example delusive means recognizing that the grounds which the person in question believes himself to have for holding the belief do not conform to normally accepted standards of adequacy. To explain his delusion, therefore, cannot be just a question of exploring the processes (e.g. in the brain) which led to him uttering the words 'That man over there is intent on killing me', but addressing the question of why he believed this without evidence and in the face of evidence to the contrary which others can plainly see.

Similarly, in the case of feelings of anxiety, there are certain norms to be taken into account, this time best described as norms of 'appropriateness'. Anxiety is intentional (again in Brentano's sense): it is necessarily anxiety *about* something, a certain kind of feeling directed towards something or some state of affairs. Someone may, for instance, be anxious about the forthcoming exams, or anxious about the threat of war, or anxious about his wife's state of health. Another person might be optimistic about the same things. Anxiety and optimism differ in what might be called their 'feeling tone': to be anxious about the exam clearly feels different from feeling optimistic about it, but no one could be described as being anxious unless they had that feeling *about* something or other. Pathological anxiety is often described as objectless anxiety, which may seem to contradict this. It would be better to describe it as anxiety about an *indeterminate* or *generalized* object – anxious feelings about nothing in particular. What makes it meaningful to call it 'anxiety' is, first, the feeling tone which is experienced, and second, the fact that this generalized feeling is realized in relation to a wide variety of specific objects. The pathologically anxious person feels anxious about everything, rather than nothing: about exams, and threats of war, and a loved one's state of health, but also about things that no one else would feel anxious about, such as going out into the open air or being trapped in a lift.

'Normal' anxiety is justified by some reasons which would be generally accepted as such in the society in question. Pathological anxiety is not justifiable in those terms, though the anxious person, in a gesture towards society's norms, may offer reasons which have more of the character of rationalizations. To explain why someone feels pathological anxiety, therefore, it is necessary to explain, not just what antecedent processes have gone on, perhaps in their brains, leading up to their experiencing that feeling; but also why they have that feeling with so little justification – why they think their alleged justifications are in fact adequate when they clearly are not. Because psychopathological conditions are, at present anyway, defined in terms of their outward symptoms, the complete explanation of why someone has schizophrenia, or obsessive–compulsive disorder, or whatever, must also go beyond the antecedent causes for the appearance of the symptoms and involve some understanding of the person's reasons for thinking or feeling or behaving in this way. Indeed, some mental disorders are standardly explained in terms of the sufferer's responses to his or her social environment, as when a 'prolonged depressive reaction' is said in ICD-10 to be a 'response to a prolonged exposure to a stressful situation' (World Health Organization 1992: 151).

These considerations are not relevant to the explanation of the symptoms of bodily disease. To explain why a rash appears on someone's skin, or why they have a headache, or stomach cramps, it is clearly not necessary to explain what reasons they have for experiencing these things. They do not necessarily experience them, anyway: one can have a skin rash without being aware that it is there. Even if they are aware of their symptoms, it is not important, from any medical point of view, to see what reasons they have for being aware of them, or to evaluate those reasons against certain social norms of intelligibility. We explain the symptoms completely without any need to understand such reasons: it is enough to trace the causal path from some inner pathological condition to the outward manifestations in the symptom. The inner pathological condition is in turn explained by its causes: we do not have measles, or cancer, or diabetes, because we have reasons to have it, but because something independent of us produces that change in the functioning of our bodies. No understanding of such reasons is therefore necessary, or even appropriate, to the explanation of the disease. The illness is not something *chosen*, but something *suffered*, caused by something external to the sufferer. There seems to be a problem, however, about saying this of mental disorder, if the above account of its explanation is correct. We are here faced with all the complex problems about mental illness as a moral and legal excuse, to be considered in Chapter 7.

Apparent differences between bodily and mental disorders

The difference between 'bodily' and 'mental' pathologies in the relation between disease and symptoms, and in the way in which we explain disease, indicates a prima facie difference in the nature of the disorder in each case. What 'being disordered' means, in the case of bodily conditions, seems to be something objective, a change in the body's functioning which is disadvantageous in some objective way: that is, in a way which is independent of the norms for judging disadvantage to which the patient themself subscribes. Being ill with measles may well be thought of by the ill person, or by onlookers, as advantageous – because, for instance, it enables her to escape some tedious engagement, or to be looked after by others, but these advantages as she sees them do not affect the description of measles as an illness. To have a mental disorder, on the other hand, is to behave, or think, or feel, in ways which diverge from certain standards held in the society to which one belongs. What counts as disordered is determined by those standards, and so may differ, as said earlier, from one culture or social context to another. To be anxious about going out in the dark because one is afraid of being the prey of evil spirits may be pathological in modern Western society, but perfectly normal in cultures which have a strong and generally shared belief in evil spirits. To believe that the man over there is an agent of a conspiracy bent on killing one may be pathological if one is a professor of philosophy who has spent his whole professional life studying medieval logic, but reasonable, and so not pathological, if one is a member of the intelligence services. In this sense of that rather tricky word, mental disorder seems to be subjective in a way in which bodily disorder is not. This is not the same as saying that the concept of bodily disorder is value-free, whereas that of mental disorder is value-laden. To say that someone is 'ill' is necessarily to make a value judgement: being ill is being in an undesirable condition. However, saying that someone is physically ill seems to be appealing to values which are not culturally variable in the way that those invoked in calling someone mentally ill are.

Mental disorder certainly causes pain or distress. At its worst, it can totally ruin someone's life, though this ruin may often be more apparent to observers than to disordered persons themselves. But is this the same kind of distress that is caused by bodily illness? Despairing about one's life, losing all sense of self-worth, becoming unable to hold down a job, or to form personal relationships – such things are at least as great harms as intense physical pain or disability, but are they the same kind of harm? They harm our relationships to the world around us, in particular to other people, whereas physical pain or disability are harms which we experience within ourselves. That is one reason why the harm which is being suffered may not be apparent to the sufferer: so that, for example, someone with a mental disorder may need to be treated without their own consent, because they do not recognize the harm as such. 'I'm not mad', as a mentally disturbed student of mine once said to me, even though it was perfectly obvious to me that (in layman's terms) he was, or at least that he was in need of professional psychiatric help.

What has been said about mental disorder could be said (with appropriate changes) about its absence – that is, about mental health. Someone can be healthy in body without feeling healthy; and concepts of what counts as physical health do not seem to vary significantly between different cultures. (Concepts of fitness may vary more significantly, but this perhaps only shows that the terms fitness and health do not mean the same thing). In both these senses, physical health is objective. Being mentally healthy does not seem to be separable in the same way from *feeling* mentally healthy; and certainly concepts of mental health do seem to vary from culture to culture: a modern rationalist, for example, might well describe priestly celibacy as an unhealthy state, but it is unlikely that priests themselves would agree. This apparent subjectivity of the notion of mental health makes it hard to see what might be meant by 'curing' a mental illness, that is, by restoring a mentally ill person to health.

Once again, proponents of neurologically based psychiatry may dismiss this distinction. It results, they would say, from an inability to free ourselves from the primitive modes of talking of folk psychology. If we knew enough about the workings of the brain and nervous system, they would say, we could define mental disorders in terms of brain disease, distinguish between this underlying disorder and its manifestations in outward behaviour, speech, expressions of affect, etc., and explain the latter causally in terms of the former. All this would be perfectly objective, and independent of any culturally variable norms. Thus, what we now call mental disorder would become indistinguishable from bodily disease: it would just be one type of bodily disease, namely, brain disease. The arguments against this kind of eliminativism have already been outlined; and anyway, we may question the assumption that whatever is rightly to be called illness must conform to the model of bodily disorder. Questioning that assumption requires us to go into more detail in our analysis of what is meant by illness, as we shall do in the next chapter.

A different kind of objection might be made to the distinction. Perhaps, it might be said, it is wrong to treat bodily diseases and mental disorders as two mutually distinguishable and internally homogeneous classes. Some conditions listed in the diagnostic classifications of psychiatric disorders do not seem to fit the criteria given above, and some recognized bodily conditions have at least some of the features said to characterize mental disorders. An example of the first might be Alzheimer's disease, where the behavioural and cognitive symptoms can be distinguished from their underlying causes in deteriorations in brain tissue, and where there are no reasons to be considered in the explanation of the condition. In these respects, there seems to be no difference from a bodily disorder like Parkinson's disease. Or we may think of the way in which such clearly physical causes as substance abuse or brain damage are manifested in ways which fit the diagnosis of mental disorder. On the other hand, such conditions as facial disfigurement, usually treated by somatic medicine rather than, or as well as, by psychiatry, might be said to be judged to be disorders by culturally variable values rather than by more objective standards. Only those who feel themselves to be disfigured (because their faces do not conform to the norms accepted in their society) suffer from this condition.

In the light of this, should we not, it might be asked, reject the whole notion of two broad classes of disease, bodily and mental, each the preserve of a particular type of doctor? Psychiatry, the argument might go on, cannot be distinguished from, say, urology in the way the latter is from, say, cardiology: the urino-genital system is clearly a different part of the body from the heart, requiring different sorts of knowledge and expertise for its appropriate treatment. But the 'mind' is not an organ or system of the body at all: it is, rather, a vague term for certain aspects of human beings. Some of the things we call mental disorders may indeed be brain diseases, others may be problems in living, others the outcome of problems in society. Lumping them together in the way we do, and assigning them to a particular sort of medical professional for treatment, may be simply an historical accident: different problems for human beings may have been grouped together in a largely arbitrary fashion, without any thought for what their real connections, if any, may be.

There is probably a strong element of truth in this suggestion, but we cannot just accept it without examining whether there are or are not real connections between the various forms of human misery we have come to call mental disorders. These connections may take the form of what Wittgenstein (see Wittgenstein 1953: Part I, para. 66f) called a 'family resemblance', rather than what he called a common 'essence'. That is, they may consist in a 'complicated network of similarities overlapping and criss-crossing', rather than in a single common set of defining attributes – but we still need to trace the connecting threads. Some may be more plausibly seen as brain diseases than others, for example: but if so, we need to see why, if at all, they may still have similarities to each other. Equally, some bodily disorders may have significant elements in common with many mental disorders: if so, we need to consider why we should still regard them as primarily bodily (or is that simply a matter of convention?).

Scientific medicine

The questions we are to consider, then, are tangled, and they are fundamentally philosophical in character. There are good reasons, as we have seen, for accepting the medical model of mental disorder – for seeing it as an illness. Mental disorders often cause pain or distress, as illness does. This pain or distress can be alleviated by drugs, surgery, and other similar medical treatments, just as they can be when they result from illness. The successful application of these treatments requires the same sort of knowledge and training which is required by medical practitioners. In all these ways, mental disorder seems comparable to the bodily diseases which would generally be accepted as examples of illness. In particular, mental disorder seems to have some kind of close connection with one type of bodily disease, namely, brain disease: many brain diseases have seemingly identical symptoms to mental disorders, and brain processes seem to be implicated in the causation of many mental disorders.

We have also seen in this chapter how there seem to be significant differences between the disorders which psychiatrists treat and those which are treated by their colleagues in other areas of medicine. The differences affect what we call 'pain' or 'distress' in the two cases, how we explain the emergence of the pathological condition, whether there are distinct disease entities, the ways in which we try to alleviate the pain or distress which arises, whether there can be anything which counts as a 'cure' and so on. These differences certainly suggest, to put it no more strongly, that psychiatry is not a standard case of a branch of medicine, as we in the modern West understand medicine.

Can we reconcile these two conflicting pictures of psychiatry and mental disorder? Only, it seems, by questioning the current understanding of what a scientific medicine involves. This kind of questioning is necessarily philosophical, since it requires us to examine some of the basic concepts by which we organize our world. What does it mean, for instance, to be 'scientific' about medicine? Does it require us to think of illness or disease or health in particular ways? Is there only one way of scientifically explaining phenomena? How can we understand the relation between mental disorder and the functioning of the brain and nervous system? We need to think afresh about the concepts of mind and the mental, of illness and disease, and of causes and explanation, and then to put our analyses of these concepts together to get a new concept of a medical model which would fit at least some of those human conditions we call mental disorders.

Medical science and modern civilization

This kind of questioning goes to the heart of how we understand ourselves in modern Western culture, for our concept of scientific medicine cannot be understood properly unless we see it as part of the self-definition of that culture: revising our concept of scientific medicine thus has an impact far beyond the narrow confines of medicine itself. In Chapter 3 and the following chapters, I shall argue that the philosophical origins of both the modern conception of medicine and of modern self-understanding in general are to be found above all in Descartes: so that a revision of that conception must involve a critique of some of Descartes's central propositions, in particular those which concern the nature of the human mind and its relation to the body. There is nothing especially new or original about criticizing Descartes's account of the mind–body relationship, but it is the contention of this book that such a critique can shed fresh light on the nature of psychiatry, its relation to general medicine, and its role in society: it can also illuminate the ethical and legal problems which arise from psychiatric practice. Perhaps this application of the critique of Cartesian dualism is sufficiently new to merit a book such as this.

The full and detailed discussion of Cartesianism will, of course, come in later chapters, but it may be a useful way of closing this first chapter and setting the scene for the book as a whole to provide a broad outline of the conclusions of that discussion. In his pursuit of a surer foundation for our knowledge of the world, to form the basis for what we should now call a scientific account of things, Descartes, as we shall see, came to separate the 'mind' or 'knowing subject' from the material world which is the object of knowledge. Thus, the ultimate outcome of Descartes's arguments was a dualist account of the world, as consisting of purely non-physical 'subjects' or 'minds' contemplating from the outside a world of purely physical 'objects' which had no element of the mental in it. Because it had no element of the mental in it, no concepts could be applied to it which made any reference to the mental: for instance, the concept of purpose, since only minds can have purposes. Thus, what happens in the physical world happens without purpose (except for those purposes, unknowable to us, which God might have had in mind in creating it). In effect, the physical world is a purely mechanistic system, in the sense of one in which one thing happens because other things have happened, and not because there is any purpose served by its happening. This system is essentially describable and explicable purely in the terms of mathematical physics. The physical world includes human bodies: so they too are purely mechanistic systems. They can be seen as machines, or automata, whose behaviour is entirely to be understood on the basis of the laws of physics and chemistry.

An important motive for Descartes in seeking to lay the foundations of a reliable science was to improve the state of medicine. His conception of the body as a machine is clearly relevant to this: it implies that disease or illness is like a fault in a machine, and that the job of scientific medicine is therefore to understand the workings of the bodily machine better, so that better ways can be found of putting these faults right. We put right faults in machines by discovering how the mechanism works when it is functioning correctly, what causes it to malfunction, and what can therefore cause a reversal of the malfunction. But Descartes's dualism also means that the mind is not part of the machine, which raises questions about what, if anything, could be meant by the term 'mental illness', and how mental illness could be put right.

In part because of philosophical difficulties about what relation could possibly exist between a Cartesian mind and matter, and in part because of increasing knowledge of the ways in which our mental and bodily lives interact, what tends to remain of Cartesianism is a dualism shorn of one its two elements: a picture which identifies the mind with something material, the brain. The mind, on this view, is as much available for scientific study as anything else in the physical world: its workings are as much subject ultimately to physical law as anything else, and to be explained in terms of those laws. Mental illness then becomes just another expression for brain disease, a fault in the mechanisms of the brain to be put right in the same way as a fault in the mechanisms of any other organ. The medical model of mental illness thus comes to be the conception of mental disorder as a mechanical fault in the workings of particular systems of the body. It is in this way that the problems referred to in this chapter come to suggest a need to rethink the very basis of scientific medicine, and with it our understanding of ourselves more generally. All these questions will thus need to be raised again, and discussed in more detail, as we proceed.

Chapter 2

Illness and disease

Being well and being ill

When we are in the mood to evaluate our lives, or parts of our lives, we can do so in various ways. We can ask how fulfilled we feel, how materially successful or unsuccessful, how much we have achieved, and so on. We can, and ought to, ask also how well we have done in moral terms – have we been kind and generous and decent and true, or selfish, mean, nasty and dishonest? An equally fundamental way of evaluating our lives, though one which is less subject to our own free choice, is in terms of health and illness. 'Being well' is at least as crucial to our 'well-being' as being fulfilled, successful, and in harmony with our fellow human beings. Although being ill may sometimes have its advantages – it may excuse us from work that we don't enjoy, or from appointments that we don't wish to keep, and it may attract sympathy and attention from others – nevertheless, most human beings regard illness as in itself a bad thing, and health as something good. Health is good, apart from anything else, because it is a necessary condition for being able to pursue many other goods: unless we are healthy, we cannot pursue many activities which we may want to pursue; our enjoyment of food and drink and other pleasures will be restricted; and so on.

Terms like healthy, ill, sick, well and so on are, therefore, used in evaluative contexts. Fulford (1989: 58) proposes it as an 'assumption' that 'the central use of "illness" … is to express a (negative) value-judgement' – an assumption which he then seeks to justify. Surely it is more than an assumption, it is a self-evident truth. We use this word and its synonyms, in everyday life at least, only when we view certain conditions negatively: to be ill is by definition to be in an undesirable condition, one deserving of help and sympathy. To be healthy is to be free of illness, and so, in that way if in no other, to be in a desirable state. The institutions of medicine exist precisely because we find illness undesirable and wish to preserve our health, or to be restored to health when we fall ill.

If we are to say whether mental disorders are illnesses in anything more than a metaphorical sense, then we obviously need to be clearer about what we mean by calling some condition an illness. Mental disorders certainly have undesirable effects on the lives of those who suffer from them, but is their undesirability of the right kind to justify us in calling them illnesses? Are the ways in which we seek to help those in these undesirable conditions comparable to the *medical* ways in which we seek to help those with illnesses? Asking what we mean by the term illness, however, raises the prior question of how we can *decide* what such a term means. In the case of a technical term, specially and consciously introduced into a particular discipline, such as 'schizophrenia', we can refer to the explicit definition of the expression, and reject as incorrect or a misuse, for example, the popular sense of schizophrenic as meaning 'in two minds'. Or we might simply say in such a case that we should distinguish the popular from the technical sense, and be careful to use each in its proper context. Is illness a technical term in the same way, or perhaps a term which has come to have a precise technical meaning? How about 'health'? If these words do have a technical meaning, ought we to use that meaning in professional technical contexts, and to reject the more popular usage as misleading? And what is the technical meaning? Does it give some kind of priority to physical or bodily health and illness? This whole tangle of interrelated questions needs to be tackled if we are to advance in our understanding of the concept of mental disorder.

Szasz, Boorse and Kendall

The anti-psychiatry movement, which probably reached its peak in the 1960s, was mentioned in the first chapter. It had various motivations, the most important of which was scepticism about the treatment of mental disorders as illnesses. One of the anti-psychiatrists referred to was Thomas Szasz, who, as we saw earlier, described the idea of mental illness as a myth largely on the grounds that the term 'illness' could only properly be applied to bodily conditions. An illness, according to him, was a deviation from the 'anatomic and genetic norms' of bodily functioning: mental disorders were not deviations from these norms, and so it was misleading to apply the term illness to them. 'I hold', he says, 'that bodily illness stands in the same relation to mental illness as a defective television receiver stands to an objectionable television programme' (Szasz 1972: 11).

Other philosophers and psychiatrists who were not connected with the anti-psychiatry movement (and even some who were opposed to it) started from the same premise. For instance, one of the most widely quoted philosophers writing about the concepts of health and illness, Christopher Boorse, in articles published in the 1970s, argued that 'the idea of health ought to be analyzed by reference to physiological medicine alone' (Boorse 1989: 90).

That is, he took what he believed to be the usage of terms like health and illness in modern bodily medicine, based on a developed science of physiology, as the basis for his analysis. He went on, 'it is a mistake to view physical and mental health as equally well-entrenched species of a single conceptual genus' (loc. cit.). That is, the primary reference of 'health' is to a *physical* condition, so that any use of it in relation to human *psychology* is at best derivative and at worst suspect. His argument for this is that 'In most aspects, our institutions of mental health are recent off-shoots from physiological medicine' (loc. cit.).

This is a curious argument in a number of respects. First, it takes for granted that the technical use of health and related terms is prior to their use in more everyday contexts, in the sense that analysis of the technical use will provide us with a better understanding of the real meaning of these terms. This assumption is highly questionable. On the one hand, these terms were in common use long before the development of modern scientific medicine, and are still in use, and fully understood, in non-technical contexts, and in cultures where modern scientific medicine is not practised. On the other, and yet more tellingly, the development of modern scientific medicine itself presupposes a pre-scientific understanding of what these terms mean. Medicine has developed as it has because of a desire for more effective ways of preserving and restoring health, which implies that we all already understood what was meant by the health that was to be preserved or restored. Merleau-Ponty, a philosopher who figures prominently in this book (see especially Chapters 4 and 5) uses the example of the relation between a map, which depicts a countryside through abstract symbols, and our experience of finding our way around a terrain. It is only the latter experience which enables us to understand the abstract symbols, so in that sense our lay understanding must be prior to the technical schematizations of science (see Merleau-Ponty 2002: x). This is surely also how we should regard the relation between the technical and the everyday uses of terms like health and illness.

Second, Boorse compounds the error. To the assumption of the superiority of technical over ordinary usage he adds an even more questionable assumption: that the historical priority of the institutions and practices of physiological over those of psychological medicine implies the logical priority of the former's concepts. It is true, as he says, that modern psychiatry developed later than modern bodily medicine, and models itself (as was said at the beginning of the first chapter) on the latter, but that does not imply that it must model its concepts, including those of illness and health, on those of physiological medicine. There is a certain circularity here. It can only be right for psychiatry to model itself on bodily medicine if its concepts are derivative from those of the latter, but the concepts of psychiatry are derivative from those of bodily medicine only if it is right for the former to model itself on the latter.

Having made the twin assumptions that the technical use of terms like 'health' or 'illness' is superior material for analysis than their use in more popular contexts, and that the historical priority of physiological medicine over psychological implies the logical priority of the former's concepts, it is relatively easy for Boorse to draw sceptical conclusions, similar to, though not as exaggerated as, Szasz's, about the idea of mental illness. 'It seems doubtful,' he says, 'that on any construal mental illness will ever be... "just like any other illness"' (Boorse 1989: 96). To reach this conclusion he also needs, as I shall argue, to make another assumption, namely, that there is something called 'descriptive' meaning, and something called 'evaluative' meaning, and that the two are logically separate. This assumption I shall seek to show to be equally questionable: but first I must set out Boorse's argument in more detail. At the end of the chapter, I shall try to show the central importance of Boorse's style of argument and its presuppositions to the overall theme of this book.

Boorse (1989: 90) distinguishes between what he calls a 'theoretical' notion of health, in which, he says, it is the opposite of disease, and a 'practical' notion, in which it is the opposite of illness. He clearly gives preference to the theoretical notion, which he says is 'value-free' (the theoretical notion is presumably preferred, though this is not made explicit, because it is the concept used in scientifically developed physiological medicine). His argument for the value-freedom of the technical notion of health takes up most of the paper cited here. 'Health', he claims, would be generally agreed to be equivalent to 'normality', but as he rightly recognizes, there can be different kinds of norms, and so correspondingly different sorts of normality. One kind of norm, as he says, is statistical: the normal is what is found in most cases of the relevant sort, but this cannot be the kind of normality we are referring to when we say that being healthy is being normal. There is no contradiction in saying that all, or most, people are unhealthy; and there are many deviations from the statistical norm which are not at all unhealthy – as in the super-fit athlete, who deviates from the norm but is still far from being ill.

Another kind of norm is what Boorse calls those 'determined by acts of evaluation': that seems to mean norms used in making value judgements, norms of desirability and its opposite. The 'standard view' of health, as Boorse calls it, is that it is these evaluative norms by which health is defined (this is the view he calls 'normativism'). Thus, for the normativist, 'to call a condition unhealthy is to condemn it' (Boorse 1989: 90). Boorse distinguishes two forms of normativism, which he calls 'strong' and 'weak'. For the strong normativist, judgements of health are purely evaluative and without descriptive meaning: this he argues, rightly, is demonstrably false (I shall return to this point later). Weak normativism allows health judgements a descriptive as well as an evaluative 'component' (what exactly he means by a component is far from clear – another point to be returned to later in the chapter). Although weak normativism is not so obviously false as the strong version, however, Boorse claims there are many counter-examples to it. Describing something as a disease, he argues, does not require one first to do an empirical survey of human preferences, and words like healthy and diseased can be applied to plants and non-human animals, where there is no question (certainly in the case of plants) of the diseased organism finding its condition undesirable.

The apparent attractions of normativism can be accounted for, Boorse argues, if we recognize that health is 'a descriptively definable property which is usually valuable' (Boorse 1989: 92). He compares it to such properties as intelligence or logical validity, both of which can be defined, he claims, in a value-free way, but both of which are usually thought to be good things. In saying that someone is intelligent, or that an argument is valid, we are not, in his view, either praising or condemning the person or argument: we are simply commenting, in the one case, on the person's intellectual capacities, and in the other on the relation between premises and conclusion in the argument. In psychology and logic, therefore, we use these terms in a purely descriptive fashion; and the fact that in other, more practical, spheres we use these terms in passing judgement on people and things is irrelevant to their meaning. The same is true, Boorse would say, of calling a person, a cat or a tree healthy: in some contexts, this might be part of an evaluation, but that does not imply that this evaluation is part of the *meaning* of the term. For the purposes of theoretical medicine, all that needs to be considered is the purely descriptive meaning.

So what is this purely descriptive meaning? As a purely theoretical notion, Boorse claims, health is the opposite of disease, which is a *biological*, not an *ethical*, concept, applying to organisms of any species. To be healthy is to be normal, in the sense of being 'that which functions in accordance with its design' (Boorse 1989: 93). The word design might seem to imply some kind of evaluative notions (something like 'satisfying the purposes of its designer' or 'fit for purpose'), but Boorse rejects that interpretation. Design, he says, simply refers to the coordination of the different parts of the organism required for the pursuit of those goals which it happens to have. The 'natural function' of any part of the organism is thus its 'standard causal contribution to a goal actually pursued by the organism' (Boorse 1989: 93). What this suggests is that to say that the natural function of the kidneys is to eliminate waste products from the organism is to say that one of the organism's purposes is to be free of waste, and that the kidneys make a central causal contribution to that purpose. Then the natural function of the parts of the kidneys is to contribute causally to the whole kidney's function, and so on. An organism is healthy to the extent that its parts are contributing causally to its pursuit of its goals, and each part is healthy to the extent that its contribution is effective in achieving those goals. To the extent that the parts do not contribute, or do not contribute effectively, the organism (or its parts) are diseased.

The goals pursued by a biological organism, as such, are biological rather than personal: the design is a natural one, and the normal is the natural. That is, they do not require any conscious sense of purpose: after all, a plant, which is incapable of any conscious sense of purpose, can have a natural design in the same sense as a human being. All members of the same species are said to have the same natural design: all members typically perform the same natural functions. The natural functions seem to include such things as eating, breathing, digesting, waste elimination, reproduction and so on – all those functions which must be performed if members of that species are to survive as individuals and reproduce themselves (i.e. ensure the survival of the species). There is thus an unmistakably Darwinian element to the notion of natural function as described by Boorse: the design of a species is that mode of functioning which is required by natural selection if the species as a whole is to survive.

Such key terms as 'design' and 'natural' used in the definition of 'health' can thus themselves be defined in an entirely value-free way: just as 'fittest', in the phrase 'survival of the fittest' is not a term of commendation – the fittest are simply those who are in fact most likely to survive. The same applies to the opposite of health, namely, disease. Disease becomes an interference with this natural functioning. It is unnatural only in the sense that it is either atypical of that species as a whole, or that it is mainly attributable 'to the action of a hostile environment' (Boorse 1989: 93). In either case, its unnaturalness is a matter of fact, implying no condemnation. That most people would find interference with their natural functioning undesirable is neither here nor there from the point of view of the meaning of the term disease. All that matters in theoretical medicine is this purely descriptive meaning.

What about illness? Illnesses, according to Boorse, are a subclass of diseases. A disease is called

> [an] illness ... only if it is serious enough to be incapacitating, and therefore is (i) undesirable for its bearer; (ii) a title to special treatment; and (iii) a valid excuse for normally criticizable behavior.
>
> (Boorse 1989: 94)

An illness is thus defined in value-laden terms but is at the same time simply a subtype of a disease, which is a value-free concept. This is explained by saying that 'illness' is a term used in practical contexts, to refer to those diseases which are most likely to be regarded by those who have them as undesirable.

It is the close tie between the concepts of illness and disease, and the particular account of disease given by Boorse, which creates difficulties in his eyes with the idea of mental illness. If a mental disorder is one which affects thoughts, feelings, desires, wishes, etc., then it is not obvious that there are species-typical modes of functioning of thought, feeling, or desire, in the way that there are such modes of functioning of physiological organs and systems. In other words, as we might say, mental disorders do not presuppose a category of mental 'diseases', of which they are a subclass. Boorse actually says that the 'social desirability' of having species-typical desires etc. is not nearly as obvious as that of having species-typical physiological processes, which might seem at first sight inconsistent with his determination to be value free in his characterization of diseases. The appearance of inconsistency can largely be removed, however, if we interpret these remarks in the following way. If the social desirability of some behaviour is determined by the contribution which it makes to the interests of society as a whole, then social desirability does not mean the same as health, in the sense which Boorse wants to give that word. According to his physiological model, something is healthy only if it contributes to *individual* survival and reproduction.

This interpretation might be supported by the fact that he takes homosexuality as an example of a mode of behaviour which deviates from the statistical norm, but which cannot on that account be treated as a disease. Nor can it be treated as a disease because, in some people's view, it is contrary to the interests of society, in that it prevents homosexuals from engaging in reproductive sex, and so helping to maintain the birth rate. Homosexuality does not in itself affect the *individual's* capacity for survival, and affects reproductive possibilities rather than reproductive capacity: the gay man or woman is not rendered infertile by their sexuality, just made less likely to engage in sexual activity which has the possibility of leading to reproduction. The implication of this example is that the norms which determine social conformity or deviance, and which are invoked in describing something as a mental disorder, are not of the same kind as those which, for Boorse, determine health or disease in any sense which is relevant to medicine. Those norms are purely physiological, and are based on the evolutionarily necessary typical design of a species.

Second, Boorse contends, it is a matter for empirical enquiry whether mental disorder is 'a nearly universal environmental injury in our species'. What this seems to mean is that this is an empirical matter in that there is no contradiction in saying that almost all human beings deviate in some way from the norms which are invoked in calling someone mentally disordered, and it is equally empirical whether this deviation is caused by 'environmental injury', that is, some external factor which leads us to think or behave in these disordered fashions. We can recall that disease is said by Boorse to be 'unnatural' either in virtue of being untypical in the relevant species or in being mainly caused by 'the action of a hostile environment'. So why is this a difficulty for the view that mental disorders are illnesses? Boorse goes on to say, 'If it is, however, [i.e., presumably, if all this is an empirical matter] one can maintain the idea that serious diseases are illnesses only by abandoning one of the presuppositions of the illness concept: that not everyone can be ill' (Boorse 1989: 95). I take this to mean that, if an illness is a disease which is serious enough to meet Boorse's three conditions, and in particular condition (ii), that it is a 'title to special treatment', then not everyone can be ill, because clearly not everyone can (logically) be entitled to 'special' treatment. But if it is logically possible that everyone might be mentally disordered, then that would mean that no mental disorder could meet Boorse's specification for the concept of illness. Even serious and incapacitating mental disorders (psychoses) could not qualify as illnesses, by Boorse's definition of that term.

Third, an illness is supposed to be, by the third condition, a disease which provides 'a valid excuse for normally criticizable behavior'. The connection is easy to see in the case of physiological illnesses: they incapacitate in the sense of preventing or making it difficult to do what the person would normally want to do. To take a simple example, someone with a gastric upset may not be able, as she would normally want to do, to prevent herself from vomiting especially in socially inconvenient situations, e.g. in the street. We excuse this normally criticizable behaviour because she did not *choose* to vomit – she wanted to stop herself, but could not help it, because of her illness. But mental disorders are supposed to affect precisely what people want to do. The person's behaviour may be held to be excusable, but not because they are doing what they do not want to do, so much as because their desire to do it is itself distorted by their illness. When McNaghten (on whose case the famous 'McNaghten Rules' are based) shot the Prime Minister's secretary, he *wanted* to do so. If he is nevertheless regarded as excusable, it is for different reasons than those which excuse the effects of physical illness. He was not incapacitated from doing what he wanted to do, but is alleged to have failed to understand the full significance of what he wanted to do. Boorse says, quite rightly, that this is a much harder conception of excusability to make sense of than one based on physiological incapacity, and certainly suggests that mental disorders, if they can be called illnesses at all, are not illnesses of the same kind as physical conditions. (For further discussion of mental disorder as an excuse, see Chapter 7).

Thus Boorse, while not in the manner of Szasz dismissing the idea of mental illness as a mere myth, nevertheless comes to a more moderately sceptical conclusion. Mental disorders are certainly not, if he is right, just like other illnesses: schizophrenia is not an illness in the same sense that, say, diabetes is. This conclusion seems to follow inescapably once we accept Boorse's physiological conception of illness and disease. Others, starting from an apparently similar conception, arrive at the opposite conclusion: that many of the conditions psychiatrists treat (though perhaps not all) are, in the relevant respects, exactly like those which their colleagues in physiological medicine deal with. In effect, on this view, some mental disorders earn the right to be called illnesses by being sufficiently like bodily conditions in the way in which they impact upon our lives.

One proponent of this position is the British psychiatrist R. E. Kendell, in his article 'The concept of disease and its implications for psychiatry' (Kendell 1975). For Kendell, as for Szasz and Boorse, the primary example of illness was *bodily* illness. Starting from this assumption, Kendell analyses a number of typical examples of bodily illness, and comes to the conclusion that the essential feature of any illness must be 'biological disadvantage' (Kendell 1975: 309). Biological disadvantage is in turn defined on the following page in terms of increased mortality and reduced fertility, just as Boorse conceives of disease as a condition which negatively affects individual survival and reproduction. Where Kendell differs from the other two authors, however, is in his view that mental disorders, or at least some of the more serious examples of mental disorder recognized in the diagnostic classifications, such as schizophrenia, can qualify as illnesses by this criterion, since they do, in his opinion, have a biologically adverse effect in the ways referred to – they lead to premature death or make sufferers from them less capable of reproductive sex. Thus, as Fulford points out (Fulford 1989: 6), we have a paradoxical, and surely suspicious, position. Two authors, starting from the same assumption that illness is necessarily a biological notion, arrive at conclusions which, if they do not strictly contradict each other, are at any rate clearly opposed: one is sceptical about the existence of mental illness, the other is clear that there is such a thing. This surely gives us some reason to look more closely at the assumption.

Critique of the physiological model

Should we accept the idea that illness is to be defined primarily by reference to its use in relation to bodily conditions? What reason, if any, do we have to accept that assumption? In Szasz's case, it seems to be simply taken for granted that what we ordinarily mean by the term illness is a bodily disorder. But that is doubtful: it may well be that the first examples which spring to most people's minds when thinking about illness are such bodily conditions as measles and diabetes, but it does not follow that all we could meaningfully include under the concept are such conditions. They might well be what some philosophers call 'paradigm cases' – clear and undeniable instances of the concept – but it does not follow that they are the only possible cases. Other instances could be accepted as long as they had sufficient similarities to the paradigms, and there seems no reason why those similarities need include the property of being bodily conditions. Even if it were the case that ordinary usage confined the use of the term illness to bodily conditions, it would not follow that ordinary usage could not be legitimately extended. Any term can reasonably be given new applications if there is some useful purpose to be served by doing so, and if the extension does not create logical problems.

At first sight, Kendell's account seems as little supported by real argument as Szasz's. He seems to arrive at his definition of illness by simply taking it for granted that it must be based on the common features of typical bodily disorders. Perhaps, however, there is more to his argument than meets the eye. By picking on biological disadvantage as the key common feature of illnesses, he in a sense both justifies the choice of bodily examples as paradigm cases and allows for the legitimate extension of the term beyond these cases. For, although bodily conditions are the most likely sources of biological disadvantage, they are not the only conceivable ones. Thoughts of suicide affect our survival chances almost as much as (though less directly than), say, blood poisoning or a pulmonary embolism; anxiety about sex is as likely to make someone impotent as hormonal deficiencies.

At the same time, by picking on biological disadvantage as the essential feature of illness in the medical sense, Kendell distinguishes, as we must do, between the kind of undesirability which illness has and other kinds, such as the undesirability of poverty, or racial prejudice, or unhappiness. It sounds plausible to say that we dislike illness, and want medical help in preventing or curing it because it shortens our lives and makes us less able to function biologically (e.g. to engage in sexual and reproductive activity). To the extent that mental disorders have similar biological effects, then our reasons for finding them undesirable are like those which we have for finding bodily illnesses undesirable, and unlike those which we have for being distressed by our own or other people's racism (moral reasons), or poverty (economic reasons), or unhappiness (which just seems intrinsically undesirable). Likewise, the kind of help we seek in order to be rid of this undesirable element in our lives is the same as when we have diabetes or measles: medical treatment, rather than moral sermons, or financial assistance, or a shoulder to cry on.

Unfortunately, however, these arguments are not enough to establish the physiological model. Illness might be distinguished from other sorts of undesirable conditions by some other characteristic than biological disadvantage in this sense. Even bodily illness might not be called illness because it brought with it biological disadvantage: that might be rather the feature which distinguished it as *bodily* illness, rather than as *illness*. It is not even true that all recognized bodily illnesses result in impaired survival chances or fertility: eczema, for instance, or migraine do not seem to cause biological disadvantage, if that is what that term means. Finally, and even if these other objections are set aside, Kendell can at best extend the use of the term illness only to *some* of the recognized mental disorders – those which are more serious and where the claim of biological disadvantage seems most plausible. The question then becomes, what do we do with the rest? Is a medicalized psychiatry appropriate for, say, some forms of schizophrenia, or severe depression, or anorexia nervosa, but not for, say, agoraphobia, obsessive–compulsive disorder, or alcoholism?

This kind of distinction seems rather arbitrary, especially since similar treatments often seem to be effective on both sides of the divide. Furthermore, we should ask whether we should ignore the fact that, even when mental disorders seem most life-threatening, they are so in a more *indirect* way than bodily illnesses. It is cancer itself which kills people: depression does not lead directly to death, but to thoughts of killing oneself, which lead to actual death only when the depressive person acts on them. It is perfectly possible, after all, for someone with depression to have suicidal ideation without necessarily committing suicide.

Even though Boorse initially presents the contention that health is to be analysed 'by reference to physiological medicine alone' as a mere 'assumption', it is he who in the end goes furthest in trying to justify this assumption by argument, even if this argument is largely implicit. I shall therefore devote more space to a critical examination of his position than to either of the others. It is clear that he gives this preference to the physiological in defining health because physiologically established norms are, in his view, more 'objective': that is, they can be determined, in his opinion, by purely factual scientific investigation, without the intrusion of value judgements. There are two assumptions underlying this conception of objectivity: first, that there is a sharp distinction between facts and values; and second, that value judgements are not, and cannot be, objective. Boorse speaks of the 'descriptive' meaning of terms, which features in 'factual' statements, and their 'evaluative' meaning, which is found in 'value-judgements', and assumes that these are separable 'components' of a term's meaning. Thus, he characterizes what he calls 'strong normativism' as the view that judgements of health are 'purely evaluative' and have no 'descriptive' meaning. To this he opposes his own view that 'health is a descriptively definable property which is usually valuable' (Boorse 1989: 92): the *meaning* of the term health (and related terms like illness and disease) can be determined simply by reference to the facts, and without reference to any value judgements which we may make about being healthy.

In making these distinctions, Boorse is following a long and honourable philosophical tradition. David Hume, in the eighteenth century, argued that it is impossible logically to derive an ought-statement (a value judgement) from an is-statement (a factual statement), and this seems to be correct. For instance, it does not logically follow from the statement that capital punishment is taking the lives of those found guilty of a crime either that capital punishment ought to be condemned or that it ought to be encouraged. The premise of this argument is a statement of the definition of the term 'capital punishment' – that is, a statement of how we in fact use the term, whether we support or oppose the death penalty. The conclusion, that capital punishment ought or ought not to be condemned, is clearly logically independent of this premise: we could consistently accept the premise but not the conclusion, but the fact that the conclusion does not *follow* from the premise does not mean that there is *no* logical connection between premise and conclusion. If we oppose capital punishment, then we have to give our *reasons* for opposing it, and one of these reasons may be that it is the taking of a human life. If this is to be a deductively valid argument, we need to imply a further premise: that taking human life is wrong. However the factual statement – capital punishment is taking a human life – still plays a crucial part in the argument: if it were not the case, then, even given the moral principle that taking life is wrong, we should not have given any kind of rational support to the conclusion.

Thus, while it may be true that factual statements and value judgements are logically distinct, it does not follow that we can separate our discussions of value from those of fact. Most value judgements are not mere expressions of arbitrary preference, like judgements of taste ('pizzas are my favourite food'). Judgements of taste are, by definition, expressions of how the person making the judgement happens to feel about something: for that reason, there is, as the proverb has it, no disputing about them. We can disagree with someone else's tastes ('I don't really like pizzas myself'), but we can hardly argue about them. In that sense, tastes are neither rational nor irrational, but non-rational. And in the same sense, they are purely subjective. But most value judgements are not like that: we can, and do, argue about them.

The argument takes the form of attempting to show that, *as a matter of fact*, some object or state of affairs conforms to, or fails to conform to, what is required by some value which we share with our interlocutor. In this sense, value judgements are intended to have a certain kind of objectivity – they are supportable by rational argument, and not just expressions of personal preferences.

An illustration may make the point clearer. Suppose I want to recommend to someone a new type of vacuum cleaner. 'You ought to get one', I say, 'it's well worth the money' (a value judgement). The other person asks me why I say that, what are my reasons for making this claim. I reply by talking about how efficient the machine is at picking up dust, how economical it is in its use of electricity, how easy it is to carry about, and how well it compares in these respects, and in price, with its competitors in the market. All these arguments in support of my initial value judgement are statements of alleged fact, verifiable by empirical means. If they are not true, then I will not persuade the other person to accept my value judgement. Equally, I shall not be successful unless the other person shares my underlying value judgements – that a good vacuum cleaner is one which picks up dust efficiently, etc. In a case like this, however, these underlying values can be taken for granted, since simply to know what a vacuum cleaner is, i.e. what it is for (which is itself a matter of fact), is to know that these are requirements of a good vacuum cleaner. Nevertheless, to say that something is a good vacuum cleaner is plainly to make a value judgement. What the illustration shows, in other words, is the inseparability in our actual discourse of facts and values, and the equal rationality and objectivity of which both admit. It would be as irrational to deny that a vacuum cleaner which picked up dust effectively was to that extent at least a good vacuum cleaner, as to deny that something weighed three kilos when that was the weight shown by a reliable set of scales.

When philosophers discuss value judgements, they tend to concentrate on examples drawn from morality, or perhaps also aesthetics, but this can be misleading if it is meant to lead to a general account of value judgements. What constitutes a (morally) good human being, or a good novel or painting, is not as uncontroversial as what makes for a good vacuum cleaner: it is not so clearly irrational in the same way to differ from generally accepted criteria in the moral or aesthetic case. Human beings and novels are not so clearly 'for' something as vacuum cleaners are. So individuals and whole societies can legitimately differ in their basic values, or in the weighting which they give to shared values. This is what gives some plausibility to the position called 'moral relativism' or 'moral subjectivism' – the idea that moral value judgements are merely subjective (it would be to stray too far from our present topic if we were to examine here whether that position is as plausible as it may sound).

Boorse sometimes talks as if what he calls normativism about judgements of health implied that those judgements were essentially *moral* value judgements. His brief statement of normativism is that it is the view that 'to call a condition unhealthy is at least in part to *condemn* it' (Boorse 1989: 90). At other points, he characterizes normativism about health judgements more ambiguously, so that it is not clear whether they are supposed judgements of personal preference, which are, as argued earlier, purely subjective, or a kind of moral judgement. For instance, he speaks of two varieties of normativism: one which holds that health is what is 'desirable for the individual' and one according to which it is what is 'desirable for society'. But what does 'desirable' mean here? Does it mean 'What the individual or society actually desires'? That would be a subjective matter, in that it would depend on what individuals or society happen to want. If no one wanted a big nose, then on this definition having a big nose would be unhealthy, which does indeed seem absurd. This interpretation is supported by Boorse's later objection to weak normativism, that it would imply that writers of medical texts had to do an opinion poll or survey of people's preferences before they could classify something as a disease. But it is also possible to use desirable in a stricter sense, to mean what *ought to be* desired, whether or not people actually do desire it. If that is what normativism means, then it is not so easily reduced to absurdity as Boorse seems to think: it implies *objective* standards of desirability, independent of what an opinion survey might reveal.

So where does this leave us? Judgements of health, disease and illness are, indeed must be, based on scientifically verifiable facts (though not necessarily physiological facts). It does not follow from that, however, that their meaning can be explained in value-neutral terms. Their meaning is how they are used. We use these terms to pick out what is undesirable, but in a particular way. Poverty is undesirable, but it is not a disease: it is undesirable because it restricts people's life-chances, and often shortens their lives. It is not a disease in part because the way to tackle it is not by any kind of medical treatment, but by economic measures to raise people's income. Moreover, the causes of poverty are not natural forces, but human economic arrangements (even when people become poor as a result of, say, a drought destroying their harvest, the cause of their poverty is not so much the drought itself as the failure of social arrangements to cope with the effects of drought). AIDS, on the other hand, is a disease: like poverty, it restricts people's life-chances and increases their mortality, but unlike poverty it is caused by a virus, a natural force. It is because of its effects that we call AIDS undesirable: but because of its causes that we call in medicine, rather than economics, to try to remove or alleviate the undesirable effects, and so call it a disease, rather than, say, a social problem.

To ask whether such terms as health, illness and disease are descriptive or evaluative is a relic of an unsatisfactory (and so largely abandoned) philosophy of language, according to which a term has a meaning (stated in its definition) either by referring to something in the world, or else by expressing an attitude to something or some situation, and these two types of meaning are mutually exclusive. Once we recognize that we give the meaning of an expression by showing how it is used, we can see that this is simply not how language works. To evaluate something positively or negatively implies that we have reasons for our evaluation, and the kind of reasons required will depend on what the term used in the evaluation means. I argued earlier, for instance, that to say that capital punishment is (morally) wrong requires justification by reasons. The reasons which are appropriate will depend on what is meant by 'morally wrong'. Hence, it would not be appropriate to justify the value judgement by saying, 'Because it costs too much', or 'Because it is so ugly', but only by giving such reasons as that it involves taking a human life, or being a form of judicial murder. Only the latter justification, or something along those lines, would show that the person making the judgement had a grasp of what is meant, in our society at least, by morally wrong – but it would not follow that to say something is morally wrong is not to make a value judgement.

Boorse says, in the words quoted earlier, that 'health is a descriptively definable property which is usually valuable' (Boorse 1989: 92). It would be better to say, in light of what has just been said, that to speak of health, or someone's being healthy, is to evaluate their condition in a particular way, determined by the meaning of the word health. To say that someone's heart was healthy because it looked aesthetically pleasing would reveal a failure to understand what is meant by healthy; but to say that it was healthy because it was performing its function in the body efficiently would be entirely appropriate (whether or not it was true).

Isn't this expressing the same view as Boorse? No, it isn't: and the ways in which it diverges are worth exploring if we are concerned about the notion of mental illness. Boorse is denying that the use of health in evaluations is relevant to its meaning – that is the point of saying that its meaning is 'purely descriptive'. He treats its use in evaluations as resulting from the unconnected fact that most people happen to value it. What it *means*, according to Boorse, is 'the normal': he follows an earlier writer in saying that the normal is 'objectively, and properly, to be defined as that which functions in accordance with its design' (Boorse 1989: 93). This may well be a good definition of what normal means in physiology, which is a purely theoretical science concerned to establish the facts rather than to evaluate them. Physiological medicine, however, is a *practical* activity: it is concerned to assess the facts in the light of certain values, with a view to helping people to overcome or alleviate certain kinds of problems. It is in that context that it uses the term normal or healthy, not in the value-neutral way it is used in physiology, but to pick out certain conditions which are relevant to its practical concerns, that is, in a value-laden way. We could not explain the use of the term in the medical context except by taking into account that evaluative force. Why does the doctor say the heart is healthy rather than that it is 'functioning in accordance with its design'? Surely because that term embodies what she is concerned with as a doctor, rather than as a scientific physiologist: as a doctor, she is concerned, not just with what is in fact the case, but with whether what is the case is *desirable* from the point of view of medical interests. But whether this situation is medically desirable can be established only by taking into account what is the case, as established in this instance by physiological science. The descriptive and the evaluative meaning (if we must use those expressions) are inseparably linked in a theoretically guided practice, such as medicine.

In rejecting normativism, Boorse is essentially denying that medicine is a practical activity – treating a theoretically based practice as if it were simply a theoretical science. Modern medicine is scientific, in the sense that it is based on theoretical science: but it does not follow that its key terms, like health, disease and illness, are not primarily used to evaluate. What is particularly important about this for our present theme is that recognition of the evaluative use of these terms as primary removes the need to tie them as closely as Boorse does to physiological medicine. That the healthy is the normal (i.e. that we justify an evaluation of something as healthy by showing it to be normal) does not entail that the normality in question must be physiological. It cannot, for reasons which Boorse states, be what is *statistically* normal – what is found in most members of the relevant population. Nor can the norms invoked be moral or aesthetic: to say that someone is healthy is not to say anything about that person's moral character or beauty. It is a different kind of evaluation from the moral, the aesthetic, the economic: one connected with trying to help people with problems of a certain kind which they cannot resolve with their own resources and which have distressing, painful or incapacitating effects on their lives.

Many problems of this kind have their sources in the failure of bodily organs or systems to function in accordance with their design – people are ill because that part of their body is diseased. Still it does not follow that that is the only kind of problem which calls for medical attention, or which can be called an illness. Human beings are biological organisms which function in certain ways but they are not just biological: in describing a human being adequately, we have to mention not only their physiological characteristics, but also their ways of thinking and feeling and responding to situations, their moods, their typical desires and wishes, their capacity or lack of it for self-control, and so on. In short, human beings have mental, as well as physiological, characteristics: minds, as well as bodies. It seems at least possible that we can speak of normality in relation to these mental characteristics as well as to physiological systems, and that the norms invoked need not be either statistical or moral or aesthetic.

Furthermore, it is not obvious that the normal, in relation to what is mental, should be defined in terms of functioning in accordance with a design. Deviation from mental normality (however defined) could conceivably create problems which people could not resolve from their own resources, and which produce distress, pain and incapacity which have an undesirable impact on their lives: indeed, this is not just conceivable, but is evidently actually the case. The impact on their lives, given what has been said, clearly need not be confined to the effect of these problems on biological survival and fertility. A scientific approach to helping people with these problems would, of course, be one based on scientific knowledge, but there is no obvious reason why the science in question has to be only physiology: it might, for instance, be psychology or even sociology, either alone or in combination with physiology.

The claim being advanced here is that the physiological model of disease, illness and health originates, in part, from confused thinking about the relation between facts and values, and in part from an excessively narrow conception of what a scientific medicine could be – one which equates it with a medicine based on a scientific physiology. If we accept this contention, then we could define illness in a way which allows the possibility that mental and physical illness might be two species of the same genus, but to accept it, we must be able to show that we can give a definition of mental normality which is in some sense objective, and deviation from which creates problems causing suffering, distress or incapacity which cannot be resolved with the sufferer's own resources. Whether there can be mental illness in this sense, in short, is as much a question about the word 'mental' as about 'illness': does 'the mental' mean anything which can be sensibly combined with 'illness' in this way? Can the mental be the subject of a genuinely objective science without being reduced to the physiological? Boorse's position rests on presuppositions about human beings and about science which are widespread in modern culture, and inevitably so because their roots lie in the very foundations of that culture. It must therefore be a major concern of this book to undermine these presuppositions.

Fulford and the agency model

In a number of essays, but above all in his 1989 publication, Bill Fulford has argued against the positions taken by Kendell and Boorse, but his argument takes a rather different form from that outlined above. His concern is more with Boorse's attempt at a value-free conception of health than with the physiological model of disease and illness, though he does point out, as said earlier, the striking fact that different writers draw opposing conclusions from the physiological model. Boorse and Szasz, with different degrees of radicalism, are sceptical, as we have seen, about the whole idea of mental illness, because alleged instances of that concept do not, according to them, have sufficient similarities to the physical conditions which they see as defining 'illness'. On the other hand, Kendell, as we have also seen, starting from exactly the same assumption, sees the notion of mental illness as relatively unproblematic, at least in some cases, because these cases, in his view, share the relevant feature of biological disadvantage with physical illness.

At the heart of Fulford's argument, however, is not the suspicion of the physiological model that these considerations provoke, but a rejection of the distinction which is central to Boorse's position, that between a value-free concept of disease and a value-laden concept of illness. The disease concept (defined in terms of biological dysfunction) is taken by Boorse, as we have seen, to be logically prior to the concept of illness (defined as a subclass of diseases which are serious enough to be regarded as undesirable). Fulford's defence of the concept of mental illness is thus centred on arguments about whether illness, whether bodily or mental, can be defined in a value-free way. The danger in concentrating on this aspect of Boorse's argument, however, is that the differences between mental and bodily illness, and in their explanation and treatment, tend to be downplayed.

The distinction between disease and illness, as Fulford begins by pointing out, has little basis in the actual usage of these terms, either in ordinary language or in the more technical context of medicine. Sometimes, he accepts, there is a tendency to use one word rather than the other, and it is true that illness is more likely to be used by patients, for whom what matters is *that* something is wrong, and disease by doctors, who are interested to find out *what* is wrong (Fulford 1989: 64). But the words, as Fulford says, are often used interchangeably. However, as Fulford accepts, Boorse does not claim to be reflecting ordinary usage. He is, in effect, offering a stipulative definition of disease and illness which is supposed to be more suited for use in an advanced scientific medicine. Ordinary usage is too loose, in his opinion, for these purposes. This methodological assumption has already been questioned earlier in the chapter, but for present purposes perhaps it should simply be accepted: the argument can then concern itself with whether Boorse's redefined concepts are internally coherent and usable.

Boorse's main reason for distinguishing between disease and illness, and for claiming that disease is the primary concept from the point of view of a scientific medicine, is, as said earlier, that disease can be defined objectively, which he takes to be equivalent to 'in a value-free way'. This value-free definition of disease follows from the definition of its opposite, health, which, as we have seen, is in terms of an organism's 'functioning in accordance with its design'. Thus, being disease should mean '*not* functioning in accordance with its design'. On this view, a diseased organism or part of an organism is one which is, as Fulford says, dysfunctional. Since design can, according to Boorse, be defined in a value-free way, it would then follow that function, dysfunction and disease can be defined in an equally value-neutral way.

To speak of the design of an organism, for Boorse, does not, as has already been said, imply the existence of a designer, a conscious being who designs it. This is important if it is to be at all plausible to speak of design in a value-free way: as Fulford points out, in the case of a designed human artefact, like a car, we must be able to evaluate the design itself, in terms of its fitness for the purpose which the designer had in mind. Then the functions of the parts of the artefact must also be subject to evaluation, in terms of their efficiency or lack of it in achieving that purpose. The natural design of an organism, however, is, as Boorse puts it, a matter of the way in which its various parts contribute to 'a goal actually pursued by the organism' (Boorse 1989: 93). That is, the organism naturally has certain goals, which cannot be evaluated as either good or bad: simply, it is a matter of fact that it does certain things which achieve certain ends. This rapidly becomes a statement, not about individual organisms as such, but about whole *species*, and individuals only as members of a species. Diseases of plants or animals are always things which 'interfere with one or more functions typically performed within members of the species' (Boorse, loc. cit.). So the design is that of a species, and is defined by those things which members of that species typically do, and by so doing achieve certain species-typical ends. Disease is by the same token a deviation from species-typical functioning.

However, as Fulford shows in his analysis of non-biological functioning (Fulford 1989: Chapter 6), we must distinguish between what he calls 'functional doing' and 'adventitious doing': that is, between things which are done as part of what the thing was designed to do, and those which it just happens to do. A car, for instance, is designed to carry people some distance at a reasonable speed: things which go on in the car which are part of that design, such as the operations of the accelerator, are 'functional doings' in these terms. The fact that this particular model makes, say, a particular noise when cornering is just something which it happens to do: however irritating it may be, it is not dysfunctional (though it may, in some cases, be a warning sign that something is functionally wrong with the car). In the same way, snoring, however irritating it may be to those near the snorer, is not a disease, not a deviation from the natural design of the human body, just something which some people happen to do (though again, it may be an indication of something else which is functionally wrong, or may in serious cases *cause* some dysfunction).

To speak of the design of a species, therefore, is to distinguish things which are species-typical, in the sense of being part of what is essential to the existence of the species in question, from those which just happen to typically occur in members of the species. This is where, as suggested earlier, Boorse has to have recourse to evolutionary theory. The natural design of a species is that mode of functioning which is most likely to secure the survival of individuals of the species and their reproductive capacity, necessary for the survival of the species as a whole. Then disease is a disturbance to that mode of functioning, and so something which undermines chances of survival and reproductive activity.

Is this really a value-free conception of design, and so of function and dysfunction? The design of an organism comes to mean, not just any old way in which organisms of that species typically behave, but ways in which they must typically behave if the species is to survive. The function of any part of the organism, correspondingly, is not just any old way in which that part of the organism may happen to behave, but the way in which it must behave if it is to contribute to the survival of the organism as a whole. Thus, as Fulford says, it would make no sense to say that the function of a kidney was to *retain* waste rather than to eliminate it (Fulford 1989: 51). A dysfunctional or diseased kidney can be defined only by reference to the failure to achieve something which is necessary for the survival of the organism as a whole. But why should we pick out survival and reproductive capacity in this way? Is it not because these are goals which are not merely typically pursued within the species, but ones which we think it *desirable* for bodies to pursue? It is because we value survival and fertility that we use the term dysfunctional of organs which operate in ways which do not further these values. Dysfunctional is itself therefore a value-term, as also is disease. The terms in which we describe functions are also value-laden, as Fulford points out: 'waste' (as in the definition of kidney function) is, for example, essentially an evaluative word – not some neutral material which the kidneys may happen to remove from the system, but something which it is a good thing to remove. Boorse himself, as Fulford also remarks, uses evaluative language when speaking of disease as being 'unnatural' in the sense of being 'attributable mainly to the action of a *hostile* [my italics] environment' (Boorse 1989: 93). An environment can be described as hostile only if it prevents the achievement of some *desirable* goal.

To define disease in terms of dysfunction is not therefore, as Fulford argues, to give it a value-free or purely descriptive meaning. The analogy with 'the mechanical condition of an artifact', which Boorse sees as supportive of his account of biological dysfunction as definable without reference to purposes or values, in fact, as Fulford points out, suggests an exactly opposite conclusion. A diseased body is 'unfit for purpose' just in the same way that a malfunctioning accelerator is. As Fulford puts it,

> the conclusion to be drawn from this analogy is that such logical constraints as are placed on the evaluation of functional objects by their being defined in terms of their functions, are, after all, evaluative and not descriptive in origin.
>
> (Fulford 1989: 108)

If both disease and illness have evaluative dimensions to their meaning, then there can be no sharp logical distinction on those grounds between them: nor can there be any reason for thinking that disease must have the primary place in the language of a scientific medicine. (The argument earlier in this chapter anyway established that the terms used in a scientific medicine do not need to be value free). Fulford therefore concludes that it is wrong to think of what he calls the 'conceptual structure' of medicine as primarily factual in character: since the key defining concepts of medicine are essentially evaluative, it follows, he claims, that it is primarily evaluative. And if that is accepted, he argues that it means that the more obviously evaluative of the two concepts, namely, that of illness, is in fact prior to that of disease – this is what he calls his 'reverse view', since it is the reverse of the conventional view which sees medicine as basically a science, and so essentially factual. (None of these conclusions seem to me to follow from the earlier arguments, but I shall return to my reasons for thinking so after further discussion of Fulford's views on illness.)

If illness is an evaluative concept, what does it mean? An examination of the kinds of human conditions which are labelled illnesses in common usage shows, he argues, that their common feature is not dysfunctionality, but what he calls 'action failure'. Illness is, he says, connected with 'the experience of failure of "ordinary doing"' (Fulford 1989: 125). 'Ordinary' doing seems to mean doing the things which one can normally expect to be able to do, and failure of ordinary doing is being unable to do the things which one can normally expect to be able to do. Whereas dysfunctionality sounds like a factual characteristic of certain kinds of operations, failure clearly brings out the evaluative nature of the judgement that someone is ill. To fail implies the existence of some norm which one falls short of: but the norm in the case of illness is, Fulford says, an *instrumental* one, rather than, say, a moral or aesthetic one. The sick person is not to be *blamed* for her failure, but helped as far as possible to overcome it.

This definition of illness is, as Fulford rightly says, in itself neutral as between mental and physical illness: so it is clearly opposed to Boorse's contention that physical and mental illness are not equally well-entrenched species of a single conceptual genus. The differences which exist between mental and physical illnesses, and which lead to the kind of difficulties explored in Chapter 1, result, in Fulford's view, from a difference in the kind of action failure which they involve. The value judgements involved in attributing mental illness are more 'problematic' and hence more 'eye-catching' than those used in attributing physical illness (Fulford 1989: 153). What Fulford calls the 'constituents' of an illness are different in character in the two cases. For example, anxiety is a typical constituent of mental illness, pain of physical. There is more variation in people's judgements of the value of anxiety than in those relating to pain – pain would be regarded more or less universally as something bad, whereas anxiety, 'although commonly unwelcome, can be welcome' (Fulford 1989: 83). This means that 'the criteria by which anxiety is evaluated are less settled than the criteria by which pain is evaluated' (loc. cit.).

There is no doubt that Fulford's account is superior to Boorse's in a number of important respects. Its recognition of the evaluative nature of the concepts of both illness and disease goes along with Fulford's view that medicine is essentially involved in making value judgements (since it is concerned with human practical interests rather than the pure theoretical description of human physiology). It starts correctly from the actual usage of terms like illness, rather than from Boorse's unjustifiable assumption that an a priori conception of what a scientific medicine must be like should determine the meaning of these terms. And because of that, it does not rule out a priori the possibility of applying the term illness to mental as well as bodily conditions. Fulford also rejects, for his own reasons, the idea that dysfunctionality is the essence of disease or illness. All these contentions are distinct improvements on Boorse's account.

Unfortunately, however, Fulford's account of illness, both mental and physical, in terms of action failure is itself open to objection. He arrives at this account as a consequence of his insistence that illness is an evaluative concept, which it is, but in rightly stressing that ascription of bodily illness involves value judgements as much as ascribing mental illness, he tends to play down the differences in the *type* of values invoked in each case. The ways in which action may fail may be, and I would argue are in fact, different in each case. To say that someone is 'ill', according to Fulford, is to say that they not merely *do* not act in certain ways, but that they *fail* to do so, and that that failure is not the result of their deliberate choice (as it is in the case of a moral failure). It must therefore be to say that something is preventing them from doing something which they could normally do. In other words, the attribution of illness needs to be justified by citing the cause of their failure. It sounds at least plausible, in the case of most physical illnesses, to see dysfunctionality in the operations of one or more of her bodily organs or systems as the cause of this person's failure. But what is the cause in the case of *mental* illness, such as agoraphobia? An agoraphobic person fails to go into open spaces, as they could normally do. What causes them to fail? Is it perhaps some breakdown in the normal functioning of their brain and/or central nervous system? If so, then this would be a cause of their failure which was distinct from their own deliberate choice, and so would allow us to classify the condition as an illness. But it would still make dysfunctionality central to the use of the concept of illness, and since the dysfunctionality would be that of one of this person's bodily systems, it would still make physical illness (and physiological medicine) primary in the way that Boorse suggests.

Defining illness as action failure can only help us to give a satisfactory account of how there can be something which can properly be called mental illness if we can say how mental causes of such failure differ from physical. Does the mind have functions of its own? Or alternatively, is there a different way of explaining the kinds of failures of action which we call mental illness than of those we call physical illness? The answers to these questions will require us, as argued earlier, to investigate the concept of the mental and the relation between the mental and the physical or bodily.

Chapter 3

'Minds' and 'bodies'

Introduction

One element in the medical model, as described in Chapter 1, is that psychiatry is simply one medical specialism alongside others. Different branches of medicine are mostly distinguished by the parts of human beings in which they specialize: cardiology deals with diseases of the heart, neurology with diseases of the brain and central nervous system, and so on. Sometimes, specialisms may be defined rather in terms of the types of patients whom they treat: a particular age group (paediatrics, geriatrics), or one gender rather than the other (gynaecology). In some cases a particular disease, affecting different parts of the body, different age groups, and both genders, may be the focus, as in the case of oncology. Where might psychiatry fit in to such a classification? It is supposed to be the branch of medicine concerned with mental illness, but the different sorts of mental illness do not seem to have the kind of common essence which the different forms of cancer have. It is not concerned only with people of a particular gender or age group: indeed, it is itself subdivided into child psychiatry, old age psychiatry, and so on. That seems to leave only the possibility that it is concerned with treatment of diseases of the psyche, the soul, or as we would nowadays say, the mind, in much the same way that cardiology is concerned with diseases of the heart. The implication of this seems to be that the term 'mind' names a part of human beings, just as the terms 'heart' or 'brain' do (some would say that mind names the *same* part of a human being as brain: but this is a claim which can best be discussed later in the chapter).

The assumption that the mind is a part of the human being which can be diseased in much the same way as any other part does indeed seem to be central to the medical model as currently understood, though it is not often made explicit. In making this assumption, the medical model reveals its philosophical roots in the Cartesian revolution which gave metaphysical form to the modern scientific view of the world. In so doing, it also created the ways in which we now tend to think about human beings and their mental lives, even if we officially reject Descartes' own account. It was hinted at the end of Chapter 1 that a major contention of this book is that any attempt to think in depth about the medical model of psychiatry requires a critical examination of this Cartesian legacy, and that critique will be the theme of this and the following chapter. Thereafter, I shall try to apply the conclusions of the critical examination to the concept of mental illness, but first I must set out my interpretation of Cartesianism and its implications. Much of what follows will be familiar to those who have even a nodding acquaintance with the history of philosophy: some parts of this history have already been mentioned in this book. Even so, I think it is necessary to spell it out here in more detail, not only for the sake of those who lack this acquaintance, but also to clarify the background to some of the more unfamiliar conclusions which will be drawn from it and whose relevance to the theme of mental illness I hope to demonstrate.

The Cartesian revolution

European culture in the sixteenth and seventeenth centuries was in a state of upheaval. In religion, beliefs and practices which had been taken for granted for centuries had been called into question by the Protestant Reformation, and even within Protestantism itself there were various competing sects and groupings. Copernicus and those who followed his lead, such as Galileo, made it seem plausible that our own planet Earth was not, as had been thought, an unmoving body at the centre of the entire universe, but was simply a planet like Mars and Venus moving round the Sun and at the same time rotating on its own axis. This contradicted, if true, not only the received wisdom of generations of astronomers but also common sense: surely, we have no sense of the Earth moving beneath us, and we can *see* that the Sun moves round about us, rising in the east and setting in the west. Along with this came questioning of the old framework of thought which saw the physical universe as finite, divided into a changeable and imperfect world 'beneath' the moon and a perfect and changeless world 'above' it (and beyond that the realm where God and His angels were to be found). The idea of a natural 'up' and 'down', distinguishing elements like earth which naturally moved downward from those like fire whose nature was to move upward also fell foul of the same questioning, and with it the whole idea that we could explain phenomena in terms of their distinct natures or essences. At the same time, the voyages of exploration made Europeans more aware than ever before that their culture, its beliefs and values, was just one among many possible ways of seeing the world and how we should conduct ourselves in it.

Not surprisingly, these upheavals created, in those who knew and thought about them, a sense of profound uncertainty. What was called into question was not only the particular beliefs that had been held, but also the acceptability of the grounds on which they had been believed. Religious belief had been based on the authority of the Church and its hierarchy: scripture was part of the basis for belief only as interpreted by the Church. The Protestant Reformers rejected the authority of the hierarchy of the Catholic church: scripture alone could tell us what was true in matters of religion, and its meaning had to be interpreted by each individual believer for himself (or herself, if we are to be anachronistically enlightened). The geocentric view of the universe, and all that went with it, was based on common-sense observation: but Copernicus rejected it in the name of mathematical elegance – the heliocentric view reduced the complexity of the mathematics of planetary motion. Galileo like-wise said that the book of nature was written in the language of geometry, and only those who knew that language could read it. Finally, views about how we ought to behave were taken for granted because they were part of the fabric of European culture, of Christendom: but was it so certain that that was suffi-cient ground for accepting them, when it was plain that other people accepted quite different rules because they were part of their own distinct cultures?

So thinking people at this time were faced not only with the problem of what to believe, but the even more intractable difficulty of how to decide what to believe. Should my religious beliefs be based on what the Church said or on what my own reading of the Bible suggests? I can't answer that question unless I can somehow know that either the Church or the scriptures is the better way to decide, and how can I possibly know that?

Similarly, in deciding my views about physical nature, should I follow common sense or mathematics? How could I know which to follow? This is what is sometimes called 'the problem of the criterion'. In order to have rational beliefs about anything, we need some way of deciding which beliefs are true and which are false – a 'criterion' – but we also need to know how to pick the *right* criterion – a criterion for choosing between criteria. This process of looking for higher- and higher-order criteria can clearly go on for ever – it is in principle impossible to complete, because that would involve a criterion which does not need to satisfy any higher-order criterion to be fully justified, and that is ruled out by what a criterion is. So we seem doomed never to achieve certainty, never to know what we should believe. This is a real intel-lectual problem permanently present in human attempts to form rational beliefs about the world: but periods of crisis like the sixteenth and seventeenth centuries bring it home to people much more vividly than times of more settled consensus about what we should believe. When we do face up to it, we come to wonder whether there is any possibility of deciding what to believe about anything.

Descartes experienced the problem of the criterion, and the profound doubts about the possibility of rational knowledge which it engenders, in his own life. At an early age, he was sent as a pupil to the Jesuit college of La Flèche, in Touraine in central France – an institution which he himself described as one of the best schools in Europe. Despite the excellence of its teachers and the diligence of its students, however, the education he received there failed to satisfy Descartes. In essence, his objection was that he was given no clearly reliable way of deciding between conflicting opinions, so that it could be said for certain after applying this criterion which was true and which was false. Without such a way of deciding, how could we talk about anything as being *knowledge*? Knowledge, properly so called, is the system of rationally grounded true propositions about the world: what it requires, therefore, is some reliable way of saying what a rational ground for believing something might be. The quest for such a reliable foundation for knowledge is the leitmotif of Descartes's philosophical work.

Rationally grounded knowledge is what we would call 'science': so Descartes' problem can be seen as that of finding a foundation on which science can be grounded. This is the sense in which his work was crucial in providing a philosophical framework for modern science. The lack of a reliable foundation was the result, as he saw it, of the fact that our system of beliefs had grown up haphazardly, without any thought of finding a clearly rational basis for them. He compared our traditional system of beliefs to an old town, in which buildings were just set down as people's whims decided, and streets just wound in and about these houses. Such ancient towns, he said, were the work of 'chance, rather than the will of men using reason' (Descartes 1985: 116). In the case of a town, we never see total demolition of the old to make way for something better, 'but we do see many individuals having their houses pulled down in order to rebuild them, some even being forced to do so when the houses are in danger of falling down and their foundations are insecure' (Descartes 1985: 117). In our system of beliefs, likewise, some were accepted because authoritative people said we should accept them, others because ordinary observation seemed to support them, but neither of these are truly rational principles: different authorities may say different things, and different people's observations might lead to contrary conclusions. The foundations of the structure of knowledge are insecure. What reason requires is some way which will show us which authority to follow, or which observation to accept – in fact, something which is independent of authority or uncritical observation.

In contrast to the town-planning analogy, Descartes can see the virtue of total demolition in the case of our system of beliefs. What is the analogy to demolition in the domain of belief? As far as the opinions which he had previously accepted were concerned, he says,

> I thought that I could not do better than undertake to get rid of them, all at one go, in order to replace them afterwards with better ones, or with the same ones once I had squared them with the standards of reason.

> (Descartes 1985: 117)

This is what is usually called Descartes's 'method of doubt'. What it amounts to is that we should subject all our existing beliefs, however self-evident they may seem to us, to systematic radical doubt – in effect, regarding them as false if we can find even the slightest reason to do so – until we arrive at some belief which withstands even the most extreme doubt, and so is indubitable. Then we can use that as a foundation on which to rebuild our system of beliefs as a whole to form a reliable body of knowledge, a science. Descartes does not apply this process of doubt to each individual belief that he held, but rather to classes of belief, defined by their sources: beliefs based on the senses, beliefs based on logical or mathematical reasoning, and finally even the very basic assumption that there is an external world at all. This last, most extreme or (as it is usually called) 'hyperbolic' doubt, is possible only if we make an equally extreme or bizarre assumption, namely, that we might have been made such that everything we believe, however self-evident it may seem, was false. It seems obvious to me, for example, that I have fingers, which are at the moment typing these words: but perhaps I might be so constituted that even this belief was in fact false – maybe I don't have a body at all, maybe all that I think I see around me does not exist. Descartes expresses this as the supposition that I might have been created, not by a benevolent God, who wanted me to know the truth, but by an 'evil demon' who wanted me always to be deceived (and not to know even that I was being deceived). We can make his point without any theological suppositions of this kind: all we need to say is that perhaps our cognitive mechanisms might be radically faulty, like an imperfect pocket calculator that always gave the wrong answers.

Commentators have rightly pointed out the flaws in Descartes' argument, but for present purposes we do not need to do so, since our concern here is not so much with the philosophical correctness of Cartesianism, but with understanding what Descartes was doing and its influence on subsequent intellectual history. (Philosophical criticism will become more relevant in the next chapter.) The method of doubting whatever can be doubted is, in effect, a method of progressively loosening our ordinary connections with the world around us. We form our view of the world on the basis of our sensory perceptions of it: our eyes, ears and other senses connect us in obvious ways with objects around us. The first step in the method of doubt breaks that sensory connection. We are also connected with the world through reason: there are some things we know – for example that two apples added to another two apples will make four apples – which do not depend on sensory observation. The next step in the method casts doubt on the possibility of that connection, but both these other connections presuppose that there *is* a world of objects, and that we are part of it, that we can know that we are connected with it, and that some of our beliefs about it are reliable, even if we may not be sure which of them are. Hyperbolic doubt destroys even that certainty. So what, if anything, is left?

What cannot be doubted, however hard we try, is, according to Descartes, that we ourselves exist, in so far as we have doubts. I may doubt, say, whether I have any fingers, but I could not even doubt that unless I was certain that I had that thought ('I have fingers') and so that I myself, the thinker, exist and am having this thought. This is Descartes's famous, 'I think, therefore I exist'. The certainty of my own existence as a thinking thing is the one thing which remains to me after the process of doubt has run its course: it must do, since it is presupposed in that process of doubt itself. Having progressively cut my links with the world, the 'me' that was supposed to be connected still remains. Central to Descartes' thought, therefore, is the claim that my own existence as a thinking being (a 'mind') is independent of the existence of anything non-mental, any physical or material world. 'Mind' becomes the name of a separate 'substance' or independently existing thing from 'body', so that a human being is a composite of two independent things, a mind and a body – hence 'dualism'. (Criticism of this claim will form an equally central part of the anti-Cartesian argument to be developed in the following chapter). Putting it differently, it is a key contention of Descartes that the 'subject' of thought, the being who does the thinking, is distinct from its objects, the things which are thought about: it is non-material, they are for the most part material. And, crucially for our purposes, one of those objects thought about is the thinker's own body: in the Cartesian view, my body is for me simply one of the objects in the world, just like my computer and the table on which I see it resting – a material object, independent of my thinking self.

What makes 'I think, therefore I exist' so certain, according to Descartes, is that we can 'clearly and distinctly perceive' the connection between thinking and existing. So this can be the criterion for which he is looking: a clearly and distinctly perceived (roughly, an immediately self-evident) connection between two ideas will, as in this case, guarantee that that connection really holds, that the belief which expresses it is certainly true. So we can use that criterion to re-establish our system of beliefs on a new and firmer basis, one that will make this system a rationally grounded system of *knowledge*, that is, a science.

By means of a somewhat dubious argument for the existence of a benevolent and truthful God who created us, Descartes seeks to restore the external or objective world which had been called in doubt and the possibility of knowing it, as long as we confine ourselves to what can be 'clearly and distinctly per-ceived' of it. What this means, briefly, is that the only reliable knowledge we can have of the world of objects is what is based on clearly and precisely defined concepts. A clear and distinct concept of an object, according to Descartes, will be one which identifies its essential character – that which makes it what it is and different from anything else. What is essential to an object, he argues, is, negatively expressed, that it is *not* a subject, not part of the mind; and more positively, that it is material or physical, and what is essential to something material is *extension*, the property of occupying space, of having a position in space and spatial dimensions.

Thus, Descartes' dualism divides the world into subjects and objects, beings who have thoughts about the world and the totally separate objective world which those thoughts concern. The essence of subjectivity is, again negatively expressed, that it is non-material, not extended – it occupies no space and has no spatial dimensions; more positively, it is thought or consciousness, inter-preted broadly to include anything which we can call part of our mental life. The essence of objectivity, on the other hand, as we have just seen, is extension: what is objective can contain no element of the subjective or mental, but only such spatial and so measurable properties as length, breadth and depth. Ideas like those of purpose, or value, or meaning, include an essential reference to the mental. A purpose is a purpose of some subject, it is *someone's* purpose, something which someone has it in mind to achieve; a value or a meaning is a value or a meaning *for* someone – something which an object has, not in itself, but only in so far as someone finds it valuable or meaningful. The objective world, simply as such, and without our consciousness of it, thus contains no purposes, values or meanings: it consists simply in objects standing in spatial relations to each other. In other words, it is a purely mecha-nistic or purposeless system. The spatial properties and relations of objects can be measured and so determined in precise mathematical terms. The rela-tions in which objects regularly stand to each other can thus be formulated in mathematical laws. In effect, objective knowledge of the physical world comes down in the end to a mathematical physics from which all such notions as purpose or meaning have been excluded. To be objective about the world thus comes to be to view it in a detached way, leaving aside any subjective ideas of purpose, meaning and value, and to see it as a purely mechanistic system governed only by the laws of mathematical physics (and what can be logically derived from them).

Cartesianism and modern science

I claimed earlier that the Cartesian revolution provided the philosophical framework or scaffolding for what we think of as the modern scientific view of the world. Much of what follows owes a profound debt to the groundbreaking discussion of Descartes's philosophy in the late Bernard Williams's book, *Descartes: the Project of Pure Enquiry* (Williams, 1978). Modern science has more of an empirical basis than Descartes allows for, and has no room for the Cartesian view of a disembodied mental substance, but nevertheless there are important respects in which how we think of science still bears the mark of Descartes's philosophy. We expect science to give us an objective view of the world, by which we mean (in full agreement with dualism) an account of things as they actually are in themselves, rather than as they happen to look to some particular subject, observing them from some particular point of view. To take a simple example, our actual perceptions of whether a room is hot or cold naturally vary depending on our own physiological state and degree of sensitivity. If we are feverish, for instance, we may find the room insufferably chilly, whereas others may experience it as quite warm. Such variations in perception are clearly not good enough for scientific purposes. They are too personal, too much the expression of how one individual happens to experience the world. So we have devised instruments – thermometers – which can give a reading which any reasonable person will accept: a reading of an objective property called 'temperature', rather than of subjective perceptions of heat or cold. This comes out in some of the ways we talk about such things. Someone says, for example, 'Is it just me, or is this room very cold?', and receives the reply, 'That is just how you feel: the thermometer shows it is 12 degrees.' The thermometer, we assume, shows us how things *really* are, whereas the person is expressing only his view of how it *seems to them*, and science, if it is to be genuine knowledge, must work with such objective realities rather than with subjective appearances.

The connection of science with an objective account is undeniable. Cartesianism enters into our view of what the word objectivity means. The concept of an objective account illustrated in the preceding paragraph could be interpreted as one which would be given by someone whose view was not distorted by special individual peculiarities, such as a fever, or strong emotions about the matter in hand, or dogmatic preconceived ideas – but we think of scientific objectivity as going beyond that. An objective account has come to mean one which would be given *if we did not have a point of view at all*. After all, any individual account, however relatively unbiased it may be, is still an account from somewhere. The individual is still reporting how things seem to him or her: the reading on the thermometer is being reported by someone, and what they are reporting is how they see it. The ideal of scientific objectivity is to describe things 'as they are in themselves', not 'as they look to a reasonably unbiased observer'. This presupposes an idea of objective reality which is independent of *any* relation to an observer – an idea which the Cartesian radical separation of subject and object allows us to conceive. The world of objects, for Descartes, is entirely distinct, as we have seen, from the world of our minds: it is what it is, without connection to what we may think of it, collectively as well as individually. The scientist, as a thinking subject, stands outside the world, and so does not have a situation within it (though the scientist's body does, of course, have a position in the world). All that science needs to do, to be objective, is to describe the world in terms of clear and distinct ideas, ideas of reason, rather than in terms of how it (the world) interacts with the scientist's body, or those of other scientists. In practice, we may have to depend on empirical data, supplied by our senses, but these data need to be interpreted in terms of rational concepts if they are to form part of a genuinely objective science.

These rational concepts were, for Descartes, ultimately those of mathematical physics. Galileo, as said earlier, had said that the book of nature was written in the language of geometry: Descartes could be seen as providing the philosophical underpinning for that metaphor, while extending it to include the language of algebra and arithmetic as well as geometry (one of Descartes's major achievements, indeed, was to connect together algebra and geometry). Science, on this view, cannot be truly objective unless it aspires to the condition of mathematical physics. All science must ultimately be reduced, on the Cartesian view, to physics, despite any superficial appearances to the contrary.

In particular, getting closer to our own themes, biology must ultimately be seen as derivative from physics, and biological systems treated as a special kind of very complex physical, or physicochemical, system. If the whole world of objects is mechanistic in character, that must include those objects which we call living organisms. They may appear, to a superficial view, to be governed by other kinds of principles, appropriate to living matter: the operations of organs such as the heart, for instance, may appear to require for their explanation the use of special biological concepts of function or purpose. When we ask such questions as 'Why does the heart beat?', it seems natural to answer, 'In order to pump blood round the body'. Yet we know, Descartes would say, that hearts and bodies are just types of physical objects, and that such concepts of purpose cannot apply in the physical world. The functions of the human body, simply as such, must be 'those which may occur in us without our thinking of them, and hence without any contribution from our soul' (that is, from the part of us which thinks and reasons) (Descartes 1985: 134). So these allegedly special biological principles and concepts must in the last resort be merely special cases of physical principles and concepts, and there is no room in them, any more than in the principles of physics, for such ideas as that of purpose. The behaviour of living organisms must be explained therefore in exactly the same way as that of any other system: the heart beats because of the physical pressures put on it, and the resulting circulation of the blood is just a consequence (fortunate for us) of this purely mechanical process.

One of Descartes' motives for wanting to reconstruct our picture of the world on a more rational basis was the hope of thereby developing a more rational, or as we might say, a more scientific, medicine. The conception of biology as a branch of physics was an essential part of this project. It meant that the bodies of human beings and non-human animals could be treated as mechanistic physical systems like any other – in effect, as machines. If so, then medicine could be seen as the repair of these machines, the more effective the more it was based on a more perfect knowledge of how the machine worked. If we knew how it worked, then when one part of the machine failed to work properly, we could know what to do to restore it: just as a clock-mender, for instance, can make clocks tell the correct time again by using his knowledge to identify and deal with the fault in the mechanism which is causing the clock to stop, or to run fast or slow. It is an indication of the depth of Descartes' influence on us that this is, in essence, still how we tend to think of scientific medicine. Illness, or disease, are thought of as mechanical faults in the body (see Boorse), and the doctor (or vet) is seen as a kind of garage mechanic whose job it is to put these faults right. The difference is that the 'machines' being treated are much, much more sophisticated and subtle in their workings than even the fanciest clock or car, and require correspondingly more sophis-ticated knowledge and skill for their treatment – and the medical model to which psychiatry is supposed to conform is based on this conception of what a scientific medicine is like.

For Descartes himself, such a medical model could never be applied to the mind, and mental disorder, whatever else it meant, could never mean any kind of mechanical fault. The body was a machine, in his view, but the mind was certainly not. The essence of the mind was distinct from that of matter: it was not extension, but consciousness or thought, which occupied no space, and so could not be governed by the principles which apply to things which are in space. If we want to understand why someone thinks something, we cannot do so by invoking mechanistic principles, since machines can't think. We have instead to look for the *reasons* why that person thinks that way: for instance, to explain why Descartes accepted mind–body dualism, we have to consider the arguments which he saw as supporting that position. Are they good reasons, which would have led any rational person to believe the same? Something similar can be said about other mental operations, like desire or emotion. Why does she have this strong desire to own that statuette? Because it is just the one she needs to complete her collection. Why is he so sad? Because he is grieving for his friend who died yesterday. Both of these are reasons which would have some force for anyone – which would have some force for us ourselves, so that we can have some understanding of the individual's action.

In all these cases, the explanation of the belief, the desire, or the feeling is not in terms of the causes which make someone have it, but in terms of the reasons which that person has for thinking, desiring or feeling in that particular way. A reason-explanation, in other words, involves some idea of choice – these are the reasons which the person concerned regards as justifying the thought etc. The causal explanation, by contrast, does not imply choice: a cause is something which acts upon someone to *make* them behave in a certain way. For many reasons, this dualism has been eliminated from the scientific view of the world. For one thing, the idea of reason-explanations is regarded by many as too subjective, qualitative, and variable to be part of a genuinely scientific kind of understanding of any aspect of the world, including our own thoughts. When we say that someone wants that statuette to complete her collection, isn't that just our *opinion* – the way we, with our preconceptions, tend to interpret her behaviour? Someone else, coming from a different perspective, might well interpret her reasons differently. There doesn't seem to be any possibility of some kind of experiment which would enable us to decide between the two interpretations objectively. A scientific explanation, however, surely ought to be objectively testable, so that it can enter into the body of generally accepted knowledge in its field.

This way of understanding the dualism of types of explanation is inseparable from the general dualism of mind and body, and that too is suspect. One of the oldest and most familiar criticisms of Cartesian dualism raises the difficulty of accounting for mind–body *interaction*. If mind and body are totally separate, and governed by totally different kinds of principles, then how can they possibly interact? Yet we all know that they do interact all the time. I have the mental experience of wishing to vote, and this causes a physical event: I raise my hand. My eyes receive light rays reflected from the tomato (an event in the physical world), and as a result I have the mental experience of seeing the tomato. How can we explain these everyday transactions between the mental and the physical on Descartes' principles? The physical side can be explained by physical principles, the mental side by those of reason: but what about the interaction between the two 'sides'? There seems to be no possibility of bridging the explanatory gap, and so having a single, unified science which can cover everything which happens in the world – thought processes, physical movements, and the connections between them. The things which go on in the mind seem to be what are sometimes called 'nomological danglers' – loose ends which do not fit neatly under any set of laws which also apply to other things. (The word nomological comes from the Greek word *nomos*, which means law or principle).

Moreover, Descartes had argued that human beings were radically different from other animals, in that only human beings had minds or souls. Hence human behaviour was directed by thought and reason, whereas that of other animals was merely a mechanical response to external stimuli. The human body was in itself just a machine, but human beings as a whole were redeemed from mechanism because of their possession of a mind which worked in non-mechanistic ways. Other animals were nothing but bodies, lumps of matter, and so were simply very complex machines, like the mechanical toys which were fashionable in Descartes' time: except that, being made by God, they were much more sophisticated in their workings (cf. Descartes 1985: 139–41). They do what they do, Descartes and his followers would say, not because they possess intelligence or reason, but in the way a clock measures the time, because of the workings of its mechanism. This created another breach in the unity of science, since our understanding of human behaviour could not be connected with our knowledge of the behaviour of non-human animals.

The ideal of a unified science, without any such loose ends, thus suggests that we should abandon the Cartesian notion of a distinct mental substance, of a mind which is not part of the physical or material world. In short, Descartes's own project of establishing science on a more secure foundation, which had led him to distinguish subject from object, ended up by abolishing the subject, or incorporating the subject in the objective world. In simpler language, mind came to be seen as a part of matter, so that our mental lives could be studied in exactly the same way as our physical lives, and discoveries about our thoughts and feelings could be integrated with discoveries about the physical world, in particular, of course, discoveries about the workings of our brains and our bodies more generally. An objective, scientific, study of mental life would treat thoughts and feelings in exactly the same detached way as the flow of liquids through a hydraulic system, or the movement of a clock (or, in more recent times, the passage of an electric current through a circuit), and would explain their occurrence and character by the same laws.

Moreover, the absolute distinction between human beings and other animals could be dispensed with, and the science of human behaviour could become a part of the wider study of animal behaviour. 'Materialism' in this sense began to develop even in the century after Descartes, with such figures as d'Holbach and La Mettrie, who saw human beings as complex machines. But it became more and more entrenched as a kind of scientific orthodoxy with the increase in human knowledge about the workings of the brain, and about the similarities between human behaviour and that of other animals. The enormous expansion of neuroscience in recent years, the development of our understanding of genetic influences on behaviour, and the reverberations of Darwinian evolutionary theory in psychology, have all given greater impetus to this kind of materialism.

In the twentieth century, the philosophical expression of this kind of materialism also became more subtle and precise. One twentieth-century form of philosophical materialism is the brain–mind identity theory, associated with such figures as J. J. C. Smart and U. T. Place (see for instance Smart 1959 and Place 1956). There is not space to go into the details of the theory here (for further discussion, see Matthews 2005b), but it will be sufficient for present purposes to say that the contention is that the development of brain science will eventually show that thoughts and brain processes are in fact one and the same things, just as in the past science has shown that, say, lightning is nothing but an electrical discharge in the atmosphere. That scientific discovery changed our conception of lightning from being something mysterious, to be explained only by invoking invisible forces such as the anger of the gods, into something which formed a perfectly ordinary part of nature, to be explained by laws which applied to other things. In the same way, identity theorists claim, future science will change our conception of the mind: it will no longer be something entirely unique and *sui generis*, but an ordinary part of nature, and its doings will be explainable by the ordinary laws of nature.

Another contemporary form of materialism, in some ways more radical than the identity theory, has already been mentioned in an earlier chapter. This is what is usually called 'eliminative materialism' or 'eliminativism' (see e.g. Churchland 1981). The details of the theory, again, need not concern us for present purposes, and I shall focus only on its central contention (again see Matthews 2005b for fuller discussion). Eliminativism is so called because it proposes, not to incorporate the mind into a unified science, but to eliminate the language of mind from science altogether – in the interests of the unity of science. Talk about minds, thoughts, reasons, emotions and so on is, according to the eliminativists, simply part of an inadequate and outdated attempt at a theory of human behaviour which, as we have seen, they call, disparagingly, folk psychology. Folk psychology is inadequate because it cannot supply precise and testable explanations of the things people do: for them, according to eliminativists, we need to turn to neuroscience, and a 'completed neuroscience' will in due course replace folk psychology. (Interestingly, from our point of view, Churchland mentions mental illness as one of the things which folk psychology cannot adequately explain.) Our scientific explanations of human behaviour will then be expressed, not in the language of thoughts, reasons, motives and so on, but in terms of such things as neuron firings, neurotransmitters and the like. A completed neuroscience, unlike folk psychology, will have logical links with other areas of science, such as biochemistry, genetics, physiology, animal behaviour studies and so on, and thus will form an integral part of a unified scientific picture of the world.

Although these forms of materialism are clearly a rejection of Cartesian dualism, there is a sense in which they still bear the imprint of Descartes: so much so that they might be called Cartesian materialism. They eliminate one of Descartes's two substances, mind: but they retain his conception of mind as a *thing*, except that it now becomes part of a bigger thing called the body. The human attributes and activities which Descartes located in his 'mental substance' are now located in a specific part of the body, namely the brain. Neuroscience, the study of the brain, takes over from introspective psychology, the study of the inner self, or mind. The subjective becomes objective, an object of study just like any other, but the conception of the objective remains Cartesian. If our mental life is part of the behaviour of matter, then it can be studied in the same detached way as any other part of matter. The laws of psychology, like those of biology, become just special cases of the laws of physics, and we can understand human behaviour ultimately in mechanistic terms. At present, we may explain, for instance, the woman's behaviour at the auction by saying that she has a strong desire to own that particular statuette, to complete her collection. This, for Cartesian materialists, is at best a temporary stopgap: when we have advanced enough scientifically, we shall be able to explain her behaviour entirely in neurological terms, by reference to what went on in her brain which led up to her waving her hand in that way at the auctioneer.

Mental disorder

The relevance of all this discussion to our understanding of mental disorder is reasonably plain. Talk of a medical model of psychiatry only has any precise meaning if we can formulate a clear conception of medicine and medical care. The claim made in this chapter is that the prevailing conception of medicine in our modern Western culture is derived from Descartes (or at least was first given a systematic philosophical formulation by him). On Descartes's account of matter, all material things, including human bodies, were mechanistic systems, or, metaphorically, machines, forming part of the greater machine called the physical universe. What went on in the body was in essence the same as what went on in any other mechanistic subsystem, differing only in its purely local features. For instance, Descartes was very excited by the discovery of the circulation of the blood by William Harvey, and saw in it confirmation of his own mechanistic explanation of the flow of blood and the role of the heart, which compared them to the operations of a hydraulic system for any other sort of fluid (Descartes 1985: 134–39). That is, he looked for the explanation of blood circulation to general physical principles. That implies that the explanation of problems in blood circulation would also lie in those same general physical principles, and that putting right those problems would be akin to, say, repairing a water pump. Medical care is on this view essentially a matter of repairing faulty mechanisms, and illness or disease is the name we give to those conditions in which bodily mechanisms break down or cease to function efficiently. Boorse's definition of disease is in this way thoroughly Cartesian.

Whether this medical model can be applied to mental disorders, therefore, depends on the extent to which they fit the conception of mechanical breakdown. For Descartes himself, as already argued, it seems pretty clear that mental disorders cannot be suitable for medical care on his model. The mind, for him, was after all definitely *not* a machine, a mechanistic system. It was governed by principles other than those of physics: the explanation of why someone had a particular thought, or belief, or emotion, or desire, was of a different form from the explanation of why, say, someone had a heart attack. The latter could be explained by identifying a cause, by which was meant some antecedent event, such as a blockage of an artery, which brought about this effect, in accordance with regularities or laws which also hold in other cases (e.g. in hydraulic pumping systems), but the former could be explained only by citing the person's *reasons* for thinking, or believing, or feeling or desiring that way. The mind was supposed to be the sphere of Reason, not of Mechanism. But that meant that when and if minds go wrong, it cannot be a matter of mechanical breakdown, to be put right by repairing the mechanism. Mental disorder must also belong to the sphere of Reason: it must consist in thinking, feeling, desiring etc. in an *irrational* or 'mad' way.

An irrational belief is one for which one has bad or inadequate reasons rather than good ones, as for example someone might irrationally believe that the earth was a flat disc rather than a sphere because they thought we would all slip off a spherical earth. An irrational desire is one for an object which does not really justify being desired, or being desired with such intensity: as someone might have a passionate wish to own a piece of utterly barren and aesthetically unpleasing ground. An irrational emotion is again one which is inappropriate to its object: as when someone is terrified of a harmless spider.

Calling something irrational, in short, is making a value judgement about it, saying that it is the kind of belief, desire, feeling etc. which one *ought not* to have. That seems to imply that one has a choice about whether to have it or not, and that persuasion by counter argument is the only appropriate way to change the belief. If I believe, for instance, that being a flat-earther on the grounds mentioned is utterly mad, then all I can do by way of dealing with this madness is to try to persuade the believer of the inadequacy of their grounds. There is no faulty mechanism which is making them believe this (if Descartes is right), so that there is no possibility of changing their belief by repairing the mechanism. If the medical model is the picture of medical care as repairing mechanisms, then this is not a medical problem. We could, of course, restrict the use of terms like mad to the extremes of irrationality, rather than applying it to the more common-or-garden varieties referred to in the examples given. People's beliefs, for instance, are sometimes so completely and systematically disordered that we say they are 'out of touch with reality'. Their desires and emotions are sometimes judged by ordinary standards to be wildly inappropriate, as when someone falls in love with a wheelbarrow. But even in these cases, if we follow Descartes's line, the disorder ought to be a matter of choice: the only kind of mental disorder possible thus becomes a *moral* disorder. We might think of those eighteenth-century institutions for the insane in which the inmates were in effect punished for their condition by harsh treatments.

This is another sense in which Boorse is thoroughly Cartesian. His suspicions of the idea that mental disorder is an illness like any other arise from the apparent lack of any organic dysfunction in the case of such disorders comparable to those we find in physical disease. Szasz is Cartesian in a slightly different sense: because of what he sees as the value-ladenness of the concept of mental disorder, he concludes that these disorders are in some sense chosen, rather than suffered in the manner of bodily illness. The 'disorder' is a strategy chosen by someone to deal with a problem in living, reflecting something of what that person is – unlike bodily illness which is something which afflicts someone from the outside, which the person can freely ask someone else (the doctor) for help in removing. Laing shares this conception of mental disorder (or schizophrenia at least) as a strategy adopted by the person, though in his case it is a form of resistance to the pressures of the family and society (including psychiatrists).

The points made about this kind of anti-psychiatry in Chapter 1 can, however, be repeated and developed in this new context. The notion of mental disorder as something chosen, or equivalent to moral disorder, hardly seems to fit the actual distressing experience of those we describe as mentally disturbed, or that of those who seek to help them. Milder forms of irrationality, such as most of us fall into, are, by reason of their very universality, fairly readily intelligible even by those who do not share them. If someone has high hopes of winning the National Lottery, for example, despite knowing the astronomical odds against winning, we may shake our heads at his folly, but still be able to understand it to some degree. We too know what it is like to dream of suddenly acquiring vast wealth without any effort, but understanding is liable to fail us when thoughts, or desires, or emotions diverge too radically from the normal. If someone believes his body is made of glass (to use one of Descartes's own examples of madness), then most of us cannot even begin to see how he could hold that view. There is no conceivable evidence that could count either for or against it: indeed, it is hard to see what could be meant by evidence in a case like this. Because of this, it does not seem to make sense to see him as *choosing* to believe this. Similarly with someone who says that he is in love with a wheelbarrow: does he, can he, mean the same by 'being in love with' as most of us do, if the object of his passion is so unusual? In cases like this, we seem to lose the possibility of a reason-explanation, which is the only kind which Cartesianism allows for thoughts and other kinds of mental processes and states.

Should we therefore turn to materialism, of the kind which I have called Cartesian? A materialist sees our talk of having thoughts, desires, feelings, etc. as really referring to physical processes, in particular, processes in the brain and central nervous system. My having the thought that, for instance, Liverpool FC won the European Champions League trophy in 2005 is in fact, on the materialist view, the same as a set of neural processes in my cerebral cortex. My feeling grief at the death of a friend is, likewise, identical with the behaviour of a number of other nerve cells. To explain the having of the thought or the feeling of the emotion is thus to explain the occurrence of the relevant neural processes, and that is done, not by giving reasons for their occurrence, but by citing the causes, in accordance with general laws of neurophysiology, which are themselves in turn derivative from even more general laws of physics and chemistry. If I have different thoughts or feelings, for instance, the thought that Liverpool's victory in the Champions League signifies the Second Coming of Christ, or the grief that I might experience at the fall of a leaf from a tree in autumn, then this must therefore be explicable in the same way. There must be some difference in the workings of the mechanism of thought or feeling which explains the difference in what I think and feel. My having these strange thoughts is then no more a matter of choice than my having measles. If we regard having the second kind of thoughts or feelings as being what we call mentally disturbed, then mental disturbance is essentially a disturbance in neural mechanisms, suffered rather than chosen, and can be treated by repairing that disturbance. In effect, so-called mental disorder is really a kind of brain disease, or the outcome of such disease, and psychiatry is the application of neuroscience to the treatment of this kind of brain disease.

Thus far, the Cartesian materialist account of mental disorder seems to fit better the Cartesian medical model than the dualist version – but perhaps this appearance is deceptive. Whether it is or not depends on the validity of the materialist identification of mental disorder with breakdowns in neural mechanisms. In some cases, this has greater plausibility than others. For instance, the loss of memory in dementia seems, from post-mortem evidence, to be clearly correlated with deterioration in those brain connections whose functioning is a necessary condition for our capacity to remember. In that sense, the breakdown of brain function is a causal condition of dementia, and repair of the breakdown, if it were possible (for instance by tissue transplants), would constitute a 'cure' of at least this aspect of the condition – in much the same way that liver failure can be cured by a successful liver transplant. Why should we not, therefore, say that dementia is a brain disease in the same way that renal failure is a liver disease? A similar analysis could no doubt be offered of other mental disorders in so far as they manifest themselves as deficiencies in normal mental capacities which depend on the species-specific functioning of the brain: for instance, the capacity to control the expression of emotions and desires in violent or otherwise unacceptable behaviour, which is known to be reduced by alcohol and other drugs.

I shall return to dementia and the other conditions just mentioned later, but for the moment it must be said that, even if the analysis of them as brain diseases which has been suggested is correct, that will not show that *all* of the conditions we recognize as mental disorders, including some of the core instances of the concept, can be analysed in the same way. Not all, for one thing, consist in breakdowns in normal capacities. Take depression for example. The disorder here consists, not in being unable to do something which most other human beings can do, such as think, or reason, or control one's own behaviour, but in doing these and other things in ways which deviate from normal standards. A person with depression can formulate thoughts, but they are not the kind of thoughts that most people have – they are thoughts of committing suicide, for instance. It is possible (though some may dispute this) to have rational grounds for contemplating suicide: for instance, someone may be faced with intractable problems in their life, financial, emotional, or whatever, which seem to have no solution and from which the only escape may therefore seem to be by ending it all. Depressive persons' thoughts of suicide seem to have no such intelligible justification: but that is not because they are incapable of reasoning – they may indeed offer a justification, such as that their life is worthless. They are classified as suffering from a mental disorder, in short, not because they contemplate suicide (which perfectly 'sane' people may do), nor because they lack the capacity to reason (they give their reasons for the thoughts they have), but because the premises of their reasoning are unintelligible to most normal people. 'How do you mean, your life is worthless?', we might say to them, in an attempt to reason them out of their depression, 'You're intelligent, kind, sensitive – your life is at least as worthwhile as anyone else's.' Unfortunately, however, our ideas of worth are not the same as theirs.

If depressives do not lack a cognitive capacity, but exercise it in an abnormal way, then is there any other way in which we could equate depression with a brain malfunction? It has been suggested that depression is caused by an insufficiency of the neurotransmitters serotonin, noradrenalin and dopamine, which play an essential part in the normal communication systems of the brain. The apparent success, in at least alleviating the symptoms, of anti-depressant medications which enable these neurotransmitters to reaccumulate in the brain (SSRIs or selective serotonin reuptake inhibitors) has encouraged the belief that this hypothesis is correct. Even the more recent anxiety that SSRIs may sometimes increase the risk of suicide, while it may cast doubt on the efficacy of this particular form of medication, does not in itself refute the underlying hypothesis. It might still be, as far as that was concerned, that depression was a brain disease, in the sense that it was the outcome of a breakdown in the brain's normal methods of chemical communication.

Nevertheless, there are other, non-empirical, sorts of objection to the hypothesis. Suppose it were established beyond all doubt that, whenever someone suffered from depression, there was an insufficiency of these neuro-transmitters in their brain. Would that help us to understand any better why they suffered from depression? In order for it to do so, we should need first of all to understand the connection between these communication problems in the brain and feelings of unworthiness intense enough to make one contemplate taking one's own life. A correlation in itself does not establish a genuine explanatory connection, since it might either be a matter of chance or else might indicate that the state of mind caused the deficiency in neurotransmitters rather than the reverse.

In a case like this, furthermore, there is reason to think that, not only do we not know of any intelligible link between neurotransmitter deficiency and suicidal ideation, but that we could not establish such a link. The reason for this is the nature of what it is to think of suicide (or indeed anything else). What identifies a thought as the particular thought it is is not the brain processes which take place when formulating it, but what that thought is about. We can distinguish a thought of suicide from the thought of setting up a business without knowing anything about brain processes or brain chemistry: all we need is to know what is meant by the terms 'suicide' and 'setting up a business'. Equally, we can know whether someone's thought of suicide is or is not rationally intelligible without knowing anything about the systems of chemical communication in the brain: all we need is to share the standards of what counts as rational justification in our culture. And vice versa: we can know all about serotonin deficiency without knowing what is meant by suicide or what counts as a rational justification of suicide. In short, there is no intelligible connection between serotonin deficiency and suicidal ideation.

It might be said, reasonably, that equally there is no intelligible connection between excessive salt intake and high blood pressure. A causal connection is certainly not a logical connection. Nevertheless, excessive salt intake and high blood pressure are things of the same kind: it is possible to establish an intelligible connection between them on the basis of known laws, tracing out the chain of links which leads from a certain kind of diet (in combination with other factors) to raised blood pressure. Serotonin deficiency and suicidal ideation, however, are things of different kinds, belonging to different vocabularies, in which the terms get their meaning in different ways. What makes it suicidal ideation, as opposed to, say, thoughts of sadness, is not comprehensible apart from a grasp of the kinds of reasons which people have for committing suicide. To try to establish a causal connection between them, rather than a correlation, would be like trying to explain why a footballer had tackled a member of the opposing team in terms of the physiology of his leg movements.

An eliminativist might seek to evade this difficulty by simply getting rid of one of the two vocabularies: terms like suicidal ideation belong, the eliminativist might say, to the terminology of the discredited folk psychology, and should be replaced by an entirely neuroscientific term. Then one neurological phenomenon could be given a straightforward causal explanation in terms of another phenomenon of the same kind. However, that presupposes that what is meant by the folk-psychology term can be adequately translated into the language of neuroscience. What kind of translation could we provide? What would be the equivalent in 'neurospeak' of 'contemplating suicide'? Perhaps it might be something like, 'having one's brain in a state which is likely to result, in the right conditions, in suicidal behaviour'. But what is 'suicidal behaviour'? It cannot be simply 'behaviour which is likely to lead to one's own death', since there is a difference between suicidal behaviour and other behaviour which is likely to lead to one's own death, such as extremely risky activities. Someone who jumps into a fast-flowing river in an attempt to save someone else from drowning is not committing suicide, even though such behaviour may well lead to their death. The proposed translation would not, therefore, capture the difference between contemplating suicide and 'being willing to take risks to help others', or, for that matter, 'being careless about one's own safety'. The distinction lies not in the brain processes involved, but precisely in the *ideation*: to contemplate suicide is to have the idea or thought of deliberately taking one's own life. Indeed, one can have this idea without in any real way being disposed to put it into practice. In the light of this, it is hard to see how the language of folk psychology could really be replaced by that of neuroscience.

Conclusions

What this shows, if the argument is correct, is that mental disorders like depression are not caused by anything neurological, in the way that, say, heart attacks are caused by arterial blockage. The disorder, in other words, is not to be explained by a disease, in Boorse's sense of a biological dysfunction – the failure of an organ or system to fulfil its role of maintaining survival or reproductive capacity, or its inefficiency in doing so. Earlier, we considered other sorts of mental disorders which do seem to be causally explicable in terms of a breakdown in a neurological mechanism: dementia, for instance. But even in their case, the breakdown does not seem really to be of the kind that Boorse or Kendell (or the Cartesian medical model) had in mind. To remember one's past, or even to recognize one's loved ones, do not seem to be necessary for survival or for (biological) reproductive capacity. No one dies, except accidentally, as a result of being unable to remember the names of everyday objects, or to identify the person speaking to them as their spouse. Even if failures of memory or recognition do sometimes indirectly have fatal consequences, it does not seem to be that which leads us to call dementia a mental disorder. Rather, it is the distress caused by their failure to remember to the dementing person themselves and, perhaps even more, to those who know and love them.

The failure in the capacity is judged, not by biological norms, but by what may be called social or human norms. We need to be able to remember our pasts, not in order to survive as organisms, but in order to have a sense of our own identity and to be able to communicate with other human beings in society: to live as human beings, rather than simply as members of the biological species *homo sapiens*.

In this respect, dementia is like depression (and indeed like other mental disorders such as schizophrenia, agoraphobia, obsessive compulsive disorder etc.): they too are regarded as disorders, not because of biological disadvantage in the sense of Boorse, Kendell, and what we can call the Cartesian medical model, but because they diminish the possibility of living the kind of fully human life that most human beings aspire to. It is probably true, of course, to say that no human being lives a *fully* human life in that sense. Some degree of sadness, disappointment, frustration and loss is a feature of most, if not all, individuals' lives. But we speak of mental disorder when the extent of the unhappiness is significantly greater than that which afflicts most of us, and, perhaps more important, when what causes that unhappiness cannot be explained in any way that most us would find intelligible. That a frail old lady living in a crime-infested area should be consumed with fear about venturing out of her home, especially after dark, is something we can understand. That a young, healthy woman, living in a reasonably peaceful district of town, should be unable to step outside her front door in daylight without being overcome by panic, is to say the least harder to understand: we treat her behaviour, therefore, as a manifestation of a mental disorder, agoraphobia.

The conditions we call mental disorders are diverse in many respects: but at least the core instances of this concept, the ones which are least controversially so called, seem to have some things in common which distinguish them from bodily diseases. They are distinguished from most (though not all) bodily illnesses in that they are deviations from what I have called human or social, rather than biological, norms (where biological norms are defined, in Kendellian or Boorsean fashion, in terms of survival and reproduction). What makes something a mental disorder is not a breakdown in any mechanism, and its treatment does not therefore consist in repair of such breakdown. The treatment which is appropriate must take account of the specificity of mental disorder, in ways to be discussed in later chapters.

The difference in the kinds of norms involved also makes for differences in the way in which we understand mental disorder, which is relevant to the ways we treat it. We understand what is humanly normal in terms of what were earlier called rational principles: roughly speaking, someone is acting normally or rationally when we can put ourselves in their shoes and see why they did what they did because that is what we might have done, had we been in their position. Similarly for thought, feeling, desire etc. This is how we understand the behaviour of the frail old lady in the example. But how do we understand deviations from the norms – radically irrational behaviour? In some cases, like dementia, a straightforward causal explanation in terms of a breakdown in neurological mechanisms seems adequate. In other cases, like depression, although there seem to be correlations with neurological processes, the link between the neurological processes and the mental disorder is obscure. It does not seem to be causal: but if not, what is the nature of the correlation? How therefore can we explain the disorder?

Finally, it is important to emphasize one other difference between bodily illness and at least some kinds of mental disorder, namely, that the distress resulting from the latter, unlike the pain resulting from the former, is at least as likely to be to others as to the disordered people themselves. If someone has an ulcer, they feel the pain and discomfort: others may sympathize with them and in this way 'feel their pain', but it is the person with the ulcer who *literally* suffers from it. People with depression literally suffer from their condition, too, as do those with agoraphobia, or in anxiety states. But in some other cases, such as dementia or (in a different way) schizophrenia, the suffering may be less obvious to the person themselves than to outsiders, and in yet other cases, such as paraphilias, there may be a sense in which persons themselves cannot be said to 'suffer' from their condition, though it does inflict genuine suffering on others.

What all this suggests is that to ask whether the medical model fits mental disorders is too simple. It presupposes that there is just one medical model, defined in terms of a homogeneous class of bodily diseases, which can be compared and contrasted with a distinct, but equally homogeneous, class of mental disorders. The discussions of this chapter point in a different direction, to the conclusion that the conditions we call mental disorders have both similarities and differences with bodily disorders, and that some have more similarities and fewer differences than others. If this seems puzzling, I want to argue, it is because we are still in the grip, even the most materialist among us, of the sharp Cartesian division between mind and body as distinct things, with totally different characteristics. A different approach, of the kind I want to present in the next two chapters, may remove much of the puzzlement and enable us to think of the relation between psychiatry and general medicine in a more adequate and useful fashion.

Chapter 4

Phenomenology and Merleau-Ponty

Starting again

It is as obvious as anything can be that we cannot begin to think usefully about mental disorder and its relation to bodily illness without first getting clear about the relation of the mental to the physical more generally. My principal contention in this book is that most of the practical problems about the treatment of mental disorder are the result of philosophical misconceptions about the nature of this general relation between mental and physical. We talk about human beings as 'having minds', and also about their 'having bodies'. We say such things as that a good student 'has a better mind' than most of her colleagues, and that sounds like saying that an Olympic athlete 'has a better body' than a couch potato. The term 'body' certainly refers to a thing, with certain characteristics, including spatial dimensions; so it seems natural to conclude that 'mind' is also the name of a thing, though a different thing, with different characteristics. Our mental lives are then the lives which go on inside this thing called the mind, as our bodily lives are those which go on inside the other thing called the body. Mental disorders must thus be distinguished from bodily disorders in much the same way that, say, disorders of the kidney are from those of the heart. The only question that remains is whether the mind is something totally distinct from anything physical, in which case its disorders must presumably be of an equally unique kind, or whether it is to be equated with a particular part of the body, probably the brain, so that its disorders are disturbances in the functioning of that part in much the same way that heart disease is a disturbance in the functioning of another part.

The discussions of the first three chapters suggest (to put it no more strongly) that this picture leads only to confusion – a confusion which is practically damaging. It is surely therefore mistaken: but what is the nature of the mistake? In his major contribution to the philosophy of mind, *The Concept of Mind* (Ryle 1949), the British philosopher Gilbert Ryle (1900–1976) said it was, or was the result of, what he called a 'category-mistake' – that is, briefly, the mistake of allocating minds to one category when they belonged to another. Such mistakes arose, in Ryle's view, partly as a result of being misled by the superficial appearance of the language which we use in the relevant context. 'Human beings have both minds and bodies', while true, is misleading. It sounds like, for instance, 'Uncle Albert has both a suit and a hat'. Suits, hats and bodies are very different things, but they are all 'things' – they belong to the category of things. It is natural to conclude, therefore, that 'minds' also belong to that category, but, Ryle argues, it is erroneous to do so.

One of Ryle's illustrations of the notion of a category-mistake concerns a visitor to Oxford who does not know anything of the peculiar collegiate structure of that university. He is taken on a tour of the colleges, libraries, research institutes, and playing fields, but asks at the end of the tour, 'But where is the university?' His question assumes that 'Oxford University' is the name of another item of the same type as, say, 'St John's College' or 'The Bodleian Library': but that is a mistake. He has seen all that there is to see of the university in seeing what goes on in the colleges and other component institutions. The university really exists, but not in the way that the colleges do: it is not a building, but a way of referring to some of the things which go on in those buildings – giving lectures, holding tutorials and seminars, setting examinations and awarding degrees. Those activities are not mysterious, but they are not visible or tangible in the same straightforward way that the dimensions of a building are. Above all, they do not take place in some special kind of invisible and intangible extra building called 'the University of Oxford'. In the same way, Ryle argues, it is a mistake to think that what we call 'mental' activities like thinking, feeling and wishing take place in some special part of human beings called their minds, which cannot be seen or touched in the way that we can see and touch their arms and legs. We should think first, he argues, of how we actually use such terms when we are not doing philosophy, or trying to think theoretically in some other way about them. When we say, for instance, that a tennis player is playing intelligently, or, in other words, thinking what she is doing, we do not mean that she is doing two things at once – one in her mind (thinking) and one with her arms and legs (doing), but that she is performing one action (running about the court and wielding her tennis racket) in a thinking, or intelligent, way. It is perfectly true to say that she is using her mind in playing like this: but to say this is not to say that she requires an extra part called her mind, in addition to her arms, legs, eyes, lungs, etc. Mind refers, not to a thing or a part of a thing, but to a way in which she performs actions: in grammatical terms, despite appearances, it is not a noun but rather an adverb.

Ryle supports his claim that the dualist conception of mind as a special, mysterious entity (a 'ghost' in the 'machine' of the body, to use one of his characteristic images) is based on a category-mistake by showing the logical problems it leads to, and by showing how another reading of the true things we can say about people's minds does not involve any such logical problems. But his critique, though primarily directed towards Cartesian dualism, also has in view the kinds of Cartesian materialism which have been considered in earlier chapters of the present book. They too regard mind as the name of a thing, but treat it as the name of a *tangible* and *visible* thing, namely, the brain. Mental activities are then those which go on in the brain. Ryle rejects this equally, as he does the peculiar form of materialism called 'logical behaviourism', which equates mental activities with the outwardly observable movements of people's bodies. He does not, however, produce the same kinds of logical arguments against materialism as he does, in great detail, against dualism, and it is arguable that he could not do so, since materialism does not divide thought and matter in the way that makes Ryle's arguments possible. Instead, he contents himself with the assertion that human beings are neither ghosts in machines nor machines without ghosts, but simply human beings (I shall return to this assertion later).

Ryle sees the dualist category-mistake, as was said, as the outcome of a misunderstanding of the things we normally say in everyday life about people's thoughts, feelings, wishes, hopes, intentions, desires and so on. In ordinary use, he argues, we handle such terms as 'thinking' or 'intending' without difficulty. We know, for instance, that we are reading Ryle's thoughts in reading his book, or seeing someone's happiness in seeing her smile, and do not feel the need to say which category thoughts, or feelings of happiness belong to. Nor are we concerned to work out the relation between the thoughts and their verbal formulation, or between the happiness and the facial configuration which expresses it. It is only when we begin to theorize about the mind, in philosophy or psychology, that we go in for a categorization which has become divorced from ordinary ways of talking, and so which falls into mistakes. What Ryle fails to explain, however, is just *why* a move away from the implicit categorization of ordinary language to the more explicit kind in which certain kinds of theory engage is necessarily a mistake: why, putting it the other way around, is everyday language preferable? Ordinary speech serves other purposes than theory: so why should theory pay any attention to it? Just because theory aims to explain human mental capacities, rather than simply refer to them, it might require a concept of mind which made such an explanation possible. To explain some features of our mental life might plausibly require us to conceive of the mind as something non-physical. To explain others might lead us to prefer the language of neurons, synapses and neurotransmitters to the everyday talk of thoughts, feelings and so on.

Merely to say that in everyday discourse we talk about various activities as mental does not in itself show that for explanatory purposes we should not think of the mind as a thing.

There is another way in which Ryle's account leaves something to be desired. He implies, as was said above, that mind is not the name of a thing, but a way of picking out certain ways of performing certain actions, but his account of this way of doing things does not make it clear why we should pick it out and say that it involves the mind. It sounds from his account as if, for example, intelligent behaviour was just behaviour which varies in response to particular conditions. It is precisely this which has led many commentators to claim, despite Ryle's own protestations to the contrary, that he was a behaviourist. Variable behaviour is, after all, still behaviour: speaking about variability, simply as such, cannot be used to distinguish what involves mind from what does not. It does not seem to be inconceivable that very complex machines could be programmed to vary their responses in ways which were appropriate to different situations. Ryle asserts that human beings are not machines, but are, simply, human beings – but what is it, if anything, about human beings which makes them human, and different from even complex machines? To find an answer to such questions, which go to the heart of what we are concerned with here, we need, I think, to turn to a different twentieth-century philosophical tradition, that of phenomenology.

Brentano and intentionality

The phenomenologist who seems to me to have most to say which is relevant to mental disorder and is illuminating about it is the French philosopher, Maurice Merleau-Ponty (1908–1961). I have discussed Merleau-Ponty's philosophy at length in Matthews (2002, 2006), but in order to understand his contribution properly, it is first necessary to set it in the context of the earlier writers in the tradition, whose work Merleau-Ponty developed in his own distinctive style. We need in particular to summarize what they have to say about the meaning of the term 'phenomenology' itself, and about the central phenomenological concept of intentionality and what it shows about the nature of the mental. This summary of their views is not intended as a scholarly contribution to the history of philosophy: it may indeed be questioned by some scholars. It will, however, serve its purpose if my interpretation of what they have to say, correct or not, is of direct relevance to understanding Merleau-Ponty's account of the mental and its relation to the bodily, thereby clarifying the concept of mental disorder.

Some historical background may be useful to begin with. The founder of phenomenology, in the sense of that word which concerns us here, was

Edmund Husserl (1859–1938). Husserl began his career as a mathematician, and studied mathematics in Leipzig and Berlin, latterly under Karl Weierstrass. Partly because of his interest in the foundations of mathematics, he then turned to philosophy, attending the lectures given by Franz Brentano (1838–1917) in Vienna. Brentano was both a psychologist and a philosopher, at a time when those two disciplines were not as sharply separated as they now are. He aimed to develop an empirically based descriptive psychology, which he also called descriptive phenomenology, because it was concerned with describing mental phenomena. By the term *phenomena* (from the Greek word for appearances) he meant 'what appears to us in perception': descriptive psychology was thus the attempt to describe and analyse our immediate awareness of the world around us in perception. It was therefore concerned neither with outward behaviour nor with neurophysiology, but with our minds in the sense of our conscious experience of things. It was meant, as was said earlier, to be thoroughly empirical in investigating this conscious experience, relying like any other empirical science on observation and experiment rather than a priori reasoning.

In order to realize his project of a descriptive psychology, Brentano needed to make a distinction between mental and physical phenomena, and the way he did it had a profound influence on the thinking of Husserl, and through him on the phenomenological movement which he founded. Reviving a medieval term, Brentano said that the essential characteristic of mental phenomena was what the medieval philosophers had called 'intentionality', which basically means 'reference to an object'. Brentano argued that

> Every mental phenomenon includes something as an object within itself, although they do not all do so in the same way. In presentation something is presented, in judgement something is affirmed or denied, in love loved, in hate hated, in desire desired and so on.
>
> (Brentano, in Moran and Mooney 2002: 41)

In view of its central importance in what follows, this definition of the mental needs to be unpacked extensively. The unpacking will involve both Brentano's own explicit statements of the definition and some of its implications, with which the explicit account is in some ways inconsistent, as will appear.

First, Brentano is saying that all thoughts, feelings, wishes, desires, and so on – everything that we think of as part of our mental lives – involves a reference to something outside itself, an 'object' (which, as he says, loc. cit., does not necessarily mean a 'thing': it can equally be a quality, a relation, a state of affairs, and so on). A thought cannot exist without being a thought *about* something or other – a thing, or a person, or a state of affairs. I can think, for instance, about the book I am reading, or about its author, or about the situations it describes: but I can't have a thought which is not about *something*. Again, an emotion such as love, fear or hatred cannot exist without an object – something or someone or some state of affairs which is loved, or feared, or hated, etc.: I love Paris, I fear terrorists, I hate being in hospital. Similarly, a wish or a desire must be a wish or desire *for* something or someone or some situation: I wish for peace, I desire a chocolate mousse. And so on through all the types of mental acts and states. Each is constituted as the particular act it is by its relation to an intentional object.

Second, different kinds of mental phenomena are distinguished from each other by the way in which they refer to their objects. Believing, for example, has a different kind of relation to what is believed than desiring has to what is desired, and that is what makes belief different from desire. If I believe my cheque will arrive today, I am in a different mental condition from when I am wanting my cheque to arrive today, even though the belief and the wish share a common object (identified by the proposition 'My cheque will arrive today'). My mental condition is thus mainly my relation to my intentional object. This is one sense in which we might take the statement that the object is within the mental phenomenon (the 'inexistence', as Brentano puts it, of the intentional object): namely, that it is essential to the constitution of a mental phenomenon, to what makes it the phenomenon it is.

Third, the intentional object need not actually exist. I can be afraid of the bogy-man even though the bogy-man does not exist; I can fall in love with Natasha Rostov even though she is a fictional character in Tolstoy's *War and Peace*. Thus, an intentional object need not necessarily be a real object, one existing in the real world. Whether *all* intentional objects could be unreal in this way is, however, open to question. For instance, could 'falling in love' mean what it does unless in most cases the objects of our passion were real persons? Or, putting it differently, isn't my talk of falling in love with Natasha Rostov parasitic for its meaning on falling in love with real human beings? It is important, as I shall argue later, that intentionality is primarily a relation to the real world: that we can identify the intentional objects that our mental states and acts refer to only by expressions which get their meaning from real objects. Without this, it would not even be possible for intentional objects to be sometimes objects which do not really exist.

Even when the intentional object is a really existing thing or state of affairs, it is equally important to say, the intentional object is the real object *as experienced by someone or other*. Intentionality is a relation between a subject and his or her intentional object: thoughts, feelings, desires etc. are therefore always *someone's* thoughts, feelings or desires. The Hellen who is the intentional object of my love is Hellen *as perceived by me*: two people may be in love with the same real person, but the intentional object of their love may be different for each. Similarly, two people may think about the same real object, but under different descriptions: for instance, one may think about the US President who was assassinated in 1963 and one about the US President who clashed with Nikita Krushchev in the Cuban Missile Crisis of 1962. They would then have two different intentional objects, even though they were thinking about one and the same real person. In this sense, the world of the intentional objects of my thoughts, feelings, wishes, etc. is my world – that is, *the* world, but *as experienced by me*. But there is no reason in principle why two separate individuals could not share the same intentional object, if they both experienced it in the same way and under the same description: indeed, this must be possible if intentionality is primarily directed to the real world, the world shared by different subjects. If you and I both think about President Kennedy, say, under that description, then the intentional object of our respective thoughts is the same: we are both referring to the same person. An intentional relation, we might say, is one between a subject and an object which are distinct, but yet cannot exist without each other: the subject's states are defined by their relation to objects, and the objects are what they are in virtue of their relation to a subject.

This makes the intentional relation different in kind from any causal relation. The object that I think about is not the cause of my thought, since, first, something can cause something else only if it really exists, and intentional objects do not necessarily exist in reality. Second, even when I think about something which really exists, my thought refers to it *as I experience it*: it becomes my intentional object because of my thinking about it as I do, rather than the other way around. There is a temptation lurking in this, as we shall see, to draw idealist conclusions, in the philosophical sense of idealism: that is, to see my world as my creation and to then assume that there can be no real world distinct from my world. But, as I have already indicated, I shall follow Merleau-Ponty in arguing strongly against this, as based on a misreading of the idea of intentionality.

The difference between mental and physical phenomena, if we follow what seems to be implied by Brentano's definition, ought therefore to be that physical phenomena are those which are defined by their inner constitution, by the stuff of which they are made (matter); while mental phenomena are those which are defined by this peculiar kind of relation to something other than themselves. A descriptive psychology (or phenomenology) would then be the science which seeks to investigate mental phenomena in that sense, and the relations which hold between one mental phenomenon and others. Unfortunately, however, Brentano's account of an empirical descriptive psychology was distorted in some ways by his inability to shake himself entirely free of a more traditional approach to psychology. Philosophers in the empiricist tradition, such as Locke, Berkeley, Hume and Mill, had represented mental life as consisting in a stream of, to use their terms, ideas, impressions or sensations. These were supposed to be contents of thought, which were supposed to be observable by an inner sense, comparable to the five outer senses of sight, hearing, touch, taste and smell, and to represent the external physical objects which we perceive by means of these outer senses. Although the empiricists in many ways rejected Cartesian dualism, this division between the external world, accessible to the outer senses, and the inner world of the mind, clearly owes a lot to Descartes's distinction between mental and material substance.

If we accept this empiricist view, then the ideas which constitute our mental life are the only immediate objects of our awareness: the objects of outer sense (such as the colour of a tomato) are really only accessible to us through the mediation of the ideas which we perceive with our inner sense. We can be aware of external objects only by having ideas of them in our minds, and these ideas are the only true objects of our awareness: thus, they are the only means by which we can be aware of external objects. The image which we might think of is that of a football fan living abroad who can only watch the Cup Final in his own country indirectly, by seeing it on his television screen. This leaves open various possible views about the relation between our minds and the external world. One would be scepticism about the actual existence of an outer world at all: if we could have no direct access to it, then how could we be sure it existed at all? How can we be sure that there actually is a *real* Cup Final if our only access to it is through the images on the television screen? Another possibility was the belief that we could know of the existence of external objects, but indirectly, by inferring them as causes of the data of inner sense. Third, most bizarrely of all, we could accept the form of idealism advocated by, among others, the eighteenth-century Irish philosopher Berkeley, according to which physical objects were nothing but collections of the ideas of inner sense. For Berkeley, 'exists' means nothing more than 'being perceived by someone'. That is, what we call the material or external world is itself mental in nature, part of someone's mind – if not ours, then God's – as if, to continue the analogy, the 'real' Cup Final just *was* the images of it on the television screen.

Brentano's language, even in discussing the intentionality of mental phenomena, often betrays residues of this empiricist way of thinking. He says, for example, that we perceive mental phenomena in 'inner perception', which is 'immediately evident' and is 'really the only perception in the strict sense of the word'. The last claim is supported by the potentially sceptical, or maybe even idealist, assertion that 'the phenomena of the so-called external perception cannot be proved true and real even by means of indirect demonstration' (quoted from Moran and Mooney 2002: 43). If we follow this line, then an empirical psychology can only be, as it was for the classical empiricists mentioned above, a study of the contents of inner sense, of a mind conceived of as a kind of inner world. Each individual has access to his or her own world, but one person's world is necessarily not accessible to other persons. The intentional object would then be 'in' the mind in a much more literal sense than was suggested earlier. The thought of President Kennedy would be something internal to the mind, discoverable by introspection, and having as a part of itself the intentional object President Kennedy. Thus, the thought would not so much *refer to* its intentional object as *contain* it.

However, this conception of empirical psychology is not really compatible with that which is implied by the intentionality of the mental. In a letter to Anton Marty of March 1905, Brentano himself says, 'If, in our thought, we contemplate a horse, our thought has as its immanent object – not a "contemplated horse", but a *horse*' (quoted from Moran and Mooney 2002: 55). That is, as the doctrine of intentionality requires, the *object* of one's thought, what the thought refers to, is something distinct from thought, something not mental but external to the mind, such that you and I could both think about it. If to think about a horse were to think about a contemplated horse (i.e. to think about thinking about a horse, then it would follow logically that thinking about a horse was thinking about thinking about thinking about thinking about … ad infinitum. We could think about a horse only if we could complete an infinite sequence of thinking about thinking about etc., which is logically impossible (self-contradictory). This is a typical example of what is called an 'infinite regress' argument, which reduces the original supposition to absurdity by showing it to lead to a logically impossible conclusion. A truly intentionalistic psychology, as one might call it, could not be this kind of study of the internal contents of the mind, but of our relation, as experiencers, to the world which we experience: of ourselves as, for example, thinking about horses.

Furthermore, (and this is particularly relevant to the themes of this book) Brentano's conception of mental phenomena as objects of internal and self-evident perception seems to revert to a Cartesian equation of the mental with the conscious. If so, it creates once again all the problems with the idea of mental disorder which I discussed in Chapter 3. Most telling of all, however, is the objection that Brentano's own definition of the mental in terms of intentionality means that mental phenomena could not be special kinds of entities inhabiting an inner world, and psychology could not be a study of such entities. Instead it would have to be a study of ourselves in our referring relationship with the physical world.

Husserl and phenomenology

It was this kind of intentionalistic psychology which inspired Husserl. What Husserl sought, however, was not a new kind of empirical psychology, but a method which could make philosophy into a rigorous science. Like many philosophers in the late nineteenth and early twentieth centuries, he saw the need for philosophy to reinvent itself, to find a new role for itself in a world in which many of its traditional functions seemed to have been taken over by the natural and human sciences. Effectively, the role which he saw for philosophy was as what we might call a second order discipline (though he did not himself use this terminology). First order disciplines, like the natural sciences, are those which seek to investigate and explain the world which we encounter in our experience. In doing so, they formulate various concepts, but it is no part of their task to reflect on what those concepts mean, only to use them in their investigations. To gain a clearer understanding of what they mean, however, is, it might be argued, essential if they are to be really useful. It is here that phenomenology finds its role. It is a second-order activity of reflecting on the first-order activities such as science: it investigates, not the world, but the concepts by which we seek to understand the world. The concepts used in first-order disciplines get their meaning from our encounter with the world in experience, so the task of clarifying them consists, as phenomenologists see it, in reflecting on that experience and the ways in which it confers meaning on concepts. That is, it involves investigating the way the world is experienced by, or appears to, us: in other words, investigating phenomena. To put it differently, it involves turning away from objects to our consciousness, or experience, of them.

Husserl, as was said earlier, came to philosophy from mathematics, and his first attempts in this direction naturally concerned the foundational concepts of mathematics: his investigations were published in his first book *The Philosophy of Arithmetic* (1891). The work was reviewed by another mathematician-philosopher also concerned with the foundations of mathematics, Gottlob Frege. Frege detected in Husserl's book evidence of a serious fault, which he called 'psychologism', by which he meant the error of treating the investigation of the meaning of concepts as part of an empirical psychology. This was an error because empirical psychology was seen as the study of

inner, subjective experience, while the meaning of the concepts being investi-
gated must be objective if those concepts were to play a part in an objective
science. For example, the arithmetical operation of addition could not be
identified with a subjective mental process of adding. If two added to two
makes four, then this is an objective fact about the numbers two and four,
not a generalization about the subjective processes which go on in the minds
of most of us when we do arithmetic. It would be quite possible for most
people to get a different answer, especially in more complicated examples of
addition, but that would not change the truth of the arithmetical statement.
Reflecting on the concept of addition, therefore, is reflecting on the objective
rules for adding one number to another, not on what goes on inside people's
heads when they try to perform this operation.

The same kind of point could clearly be made about other sorts of concepts.
To reflect on the concept of time, for example, is to think about what is meant
by time: not what *I* mean by it, or *you* mean by it. The concept of time is,
for instance, what two people who disagree about the nature of time must
share, since without a shared understanding of time they could not genuinely
disagree with each other. Concepts exist, we might say, not inside people's
minds, but in the space between people, and what they mean is therefore not
to be established by an empirical investigation of people's psychology. Husserl
accepted the force of this kind of critique of psychologism, and for the rest
of his life developed a concept of phenomenology which sharply distinguished
it from empirical psychology.

Nevertheless, he still thought it necessary to relate the meaning of concepts
to its roots in the experience of subjects. What, after all, could, say, 'time' mean
except what *we* meant by it? The meaning of a concept could not, for the
reasons spelled out above, be identified with what went on inside the head of
an individual, but it could not be divorced from the consciousness of subjects
in general: meaning was given to concepts by those who used them. A
phenomenological investigation of the meaning of concepts could not be
separated therefore from reflection on the consciousness which gave them
meaning. How could this be reconciled with the abandonment of psychologism? How could we think of the meanings of concepts as being objective
while also regarding them as existing only relative to a consciousness?

Husserl's solution was to make phenomenology transcendental. Reviving a
Kantian term, Husserl talked about a 'transcendental ego' or 'transcendental
consciousness' as endowing concepts with meaning. A transcendental
consciousness is not that of any particular individual, but consciousness
as such, consciousness in general, that which all conscious beings have in
common. Consciousness in general, like particular consciousnesses, is intentional

in Brentano's sense: it refers beyond itself to its intentional objects. Thought in general, for instance, is constituted as what it is, not by its inner substance, but by its reference to something outside itself. Phenomenology, therefore, in investigating the roots of meaning in consciousness or experience, is not engaged in introspective psychology, but in our relation as conscious beings to things outside ourselves.

If phenomenology is an investigation of the roots of meaning, its attention must, in Husserl's view, be focused on the subjective term of that relation – on our consciousness of the world, rather than on the world of which we are conscious. A first-order study, like physics or empirical psychology, is directed towards the world of objects, including the human mind as one of those objects. Such studies use the concepts which we are to investigate in phenomenology, that is, they apply the concepts to objects, e.g. the concept of 'extension' to physical objects. In so doing, they necessarily make certain assumptions about the objective world: that it exists, that it is spread out in space and time, that causal relationships exist between objects and events in the world, and so on. These assumptions constitute what Husserl called the 'natural attitude': they are the assumptions which we all make, as part of common sense as well as of scientific thinking. We must make them in order to carry on our existence in the world. But phenomenology, at least as he saw it in the earlier phase of his thought, required us to take a step back from this natural attitude. It, after all, is concerned, not with living in the world but with understanding the ways in which we think about the world. So the first essential of phenomenology was to set aside ('put in brackets', as Husserl put it) these natural assumptions. Then we could consider the phenomena just as such: that is, we could reflect on how things present themselves to us in our experience, without concerning ourselves about whether they actually exist independently of our experience of them.

So phenomenology is not concerned with giving a causal explanation of what we experience, e.g. in terms of the influence of external objects on our sense organs, and the consequent processes which go on in our nervous systems and brains, which result in our experience. Rather, the phenomenologist seeks to *describe* our experience just as we have it, without making any assumptions (or 'presuppositions', as Husserl calls them) about its causes, if any, or anything outside the experience itself. We set aside the natural attitude, not in the sense that we seriously doubt whether the external world exists and causes our experiences, but in the sense that it is not part of our concern as phenomenologists whether its exists or not. We can do this because, as we have seen, the intentional object of an experience need not be a really existing object: so, Husserl concludes, we can reflect on, say, my thought about the University of Aberdeen without presupposing that there is such an institution. This bracketing of the natural attitude is achieved by what Husserl calls the 'phenomenological reduction'. To carry out the reduction is to hold back from all commitment to the real existence of the intentional objects of our consciousness in order to concentrate on consciousness itself (Husserl uses the Greek word *epoche*, literally meaning 'holding away from'). Paradoxically, however, this holding away from the natural attitude is also seen by Husserl as a 'return to the things themselves'. Phenomenological description, after all, is meant to be a description of the world as we actually encounter it in living experience, not the world as interpreted in terms of the theoretical concepts of science or philosophy. It is a return to the concrete base on which the whole structure of abstract theory is raised.

We can, unfortunately, see the roots of a problem here in Husserl's earlier conception of phenomenology. The promise of a return to the things themselves suggests that the aim of the project is to get back to a concrete realism, to human beings and their experience as the source of abstract theorizing. But the phenomenological reduction, which is supposed to get us back there, seems to consist in divorcing ourselves from concrete experience. Our actual encounter with the world is with things, not with the representations of things: this is implicit, as was argued earlier, in the whole notion of the intentionality of consciousness. It is true that intentional objects need not always be really existing things; but I suggested above that it is arguable that most of them must be. I can be afraid of a nonexistent bogy-man, only because I know what it means to be afraid of things which actually exist: how else could I know what fear meant, and unless I knew what fear was, how could I distinguish being afraid from any other state of consciousness? Being afraid is a matter, not just of my purely inner state, but also of relating to the world outside of me in certain ways: being disposed to run away from the object of fear, for example.

Hence, as Merleau-Ponty points out, a complete phenomenological reduction is impossible (Merleau-Ponty 2002: xv). If human experience or consciousness is intentional, as Husserl himself accepted, then we cannot separate consciousness completely from the world of which it is conscious. Consciousness cannot exist independently of its relation to the world – 'we are through and through compounded of relationships with the world' (Merleau-Ponty 2002: xiv). Thus, the phenomenologist cannot reflect on consciousness as a distinct domain. To attempt to do that is to fall back into Cartesian dualism, and it is significant that Husserl himself makes the comparison between the phenomenological project and Descartes' quest, in his *Meditations on First Philosophy*, for an absolute foundation of knowledge (Husserl 1960). Once we revert to dualism in this way, we move away from concrete realism, since we distinguish between the ideas or representations with which consciousness is engaged and the real things which those ideas are supposed to represent. Then, as argued earlier, the alternatives seem to be either sceptical doubt about whether there are such real things (since we have no direct access to them) or else some form of idealism, the view that ideas in the mind do not just *represent* real things, but *are* the only reality. Husserl, in this earlier phase of his thinking, was constantly tempted by the notion of transcendental idealism as implicit in phenomenology.

This is where the importance of Husserl's transcendental turn becomes obvious. If we separate consciousness from the world it is consciousness of, then we seem to be committed to identifying the subject of consciousness, the I or ego which is conscious, not with any concrete individual human being existing in a real situation within the world, but with some kind of abstract subjectivity-as-such. The first-person pronoun, as indicating a particular human individual, requires for its meaning a possibility of contrast with other Is or egos. I am conscious of the world from my point of view, and you from your, different, point of view. Each I has his or her point of view on a *common* world: we could not speak meaningfully of a point of view without differentiating it from others, and we could not differentiate it from others unless they were all points of view on the same world. We can identify something as an object of our consciousness only if others can also identify it as an object of theirs, so that we can compare and contrast our point of view with theirs. To speak of 'I' in the ordinary sense as a subject of consciousness is thus to see that I as part of the world, looking out on it from where the person in question happens to be. And it is also to accept the existence of other selves, with different points of view, also inhabiting the world. *My* world in that way becomes inconceivable apart from *the* world. If the phenomenological subject, therefore, is distinguished from the world of which it is conscious, then it cannot be identified with my consciousness or yours. It must be conceived of as a subject which is not in any particular place in the world, but, as it were, stands outside the world, looking on it without being involved with it: in short, as a transcendental ego. And there can only be one such transcendental ego: it is an I which is not part of any we. But then the question returns: how can we avoid psychologism without taking a transcendental turn?

Heidegger and 'being-in-the-world'

The problem for Husserlian phenomenology in this earlier phase thus arose from a conflict between the desire to provide an absolute grounding for all meaningful thought about the world and the desire to get away from abstract theorizing and back to concrete human experience. Both of these desires had their source in a sense that theorizing about the world took too much for granted, because it had lost contact with its roots in common human experience. In a curious way Husserl's early phenomenology, with its wish to establish itself as a rigorous science, had itself become precisely that kind of abstract theory about consciousness. Husserl's most distinguished student, Martin Heidegger (1889–1976), in his major work *Being and Time* (Heidegger 1962), saw that the conflict could be resolved only by going back to the original source and so moving away from the idea that phenomenology must be a rigorous science. We should start, not from some ideal absolute, but from where we actually are. Our experience of the world is that of beings who are *in* the world, in some specific place and time, and for that very reason, experience or consciousness is not a matter of pure intellectual contemplation, but of active and emotional engagement with the world in various ways.

Part of the reason for the tendency of both Brentano and Husserl to slide into some form of idealism is their (thoroughly Cartesian) conception of consciousness as essentially *cognitive,* as a matter of forming representations of the world. That makes consciousness primarily theoretical, as if our contact with the world was like looking at diagrams of things, while the things themselves lie behind what is sometimes called the 'veil of perception'. Then the question becomes how we can connect up these representations with what they represent, and the answer, as we have seen, is liable to be either sceptical or idealist. But if we genuinely reflect on our actual consciousness of things and people, we see immediately that it is not essentially theoretical or purely cognitive: it is practical. We handle things, and make use of them, and respond emotionally to them, before we think about them. We can only think about them in an abstract or theoretical way *because* we first handle them and make use of them. Unless we had a sense of them as independently real in this way, we could not begin to give any meaning to the concepts we form of them for theoretical purposes. The terms by which we identify objects get their meaning from their use in the common language which we share with others in the course of our common practical engagement with the world.

Heidegger expresses all this by saying that human being is essentially 'being-in-the-world'. The human mode of being he describes by using the German word *Dasein* (literally 'being there'). Most things (other than abstract entities like geometrical objects or numbers) do, of course, have their being in the world: but Heidegger reserves this term in a special sense for human beings. We are in the world in a particular sense, namely, that we are subjectively aware of it. My computer is in the world in the sense that it has a particular location in space (on my desk, in my study) and time (it was produced at some time in the past, is now in front of me as I work on it), and has causal relations with the objects round it, including me (light from the window plays on it, and the reflected light reaches my eyes and affects my retina; I type these words by depressing the keys on the keyboard, and so on). But none of these ways of being involve the computer's awareness, since it has no such thing. I too have this kind of relationship with objects in the world, because in some ways I too am an object. I too have a place in space and time (now, sitting at my desk in my study). Things around me have a causal impact on me. But in addition to being an object, I am also in the world as a subject, as a being who also has the kinds of relationship to objects which involves awareness. I am pressing the computer keys as part of my plan to write this book, and I am reading the words on the screen as part of the same plan.

Describing human being as being-in-the-world (which is a single word in German, *Inderweltsein*) is saying that human beings exist both as subjects and as objects, and further that our subjectivity and our objectivity are inseparably linked. Because we are objects in the world, and therefore have a position in space and time and characteristics derived from the causal influence of other objects on us, our subjectivity is necessarily perspectival. That is, we are aware of the world always from a certain point of view, determined by our spatiotemporal position and our causally influenced characteristics. Thus, (if I may personalize by way of illustration) my perspective at the moment is from my chair at my desk, where I am now sitting, and it is that of a white male of pensionable age, married and with two children, whose main occupation in life has been as an academic philosopher, etc. etc. But because we are subjects, the objects of which we are aware are objects as seen by us from our perspective, not objects which we contemplate in a detached and dispassionate fashion. I am aware of my desk, for instance, not simply as a rectangular topped black wooden thing on which rest other things of different shapes, sizes and materials, but as *my desk*. It is where I do a lot of my work, and have done other pieces of work in the past. The objects on it are my computer, with its screen and printer, which I use for my writing; a telephone, which I use to speak to family, friends, colleagues and others; and books and papers, which I can consult in the course of my writing. The world of objects is not value- and meaning-free, but charged with meaning for me.

Being-in-the-world in the way human beings are is thus not simply a matter of being one object amongst others: it is being actively engaged in the world, in ways which make other objects meaningful to us. Equally, it clearly is not being a detached Cartesian subject, contemplating the world of objects from outside, through the intermediary of representations or ideas – somewhat in the way, to repeat the image used already, that we might view the Cup Final from afar on the television screen. Human being is being there, being in the stadium and participating to some extent at least in the action. The Cartesian view of the relation between subject and object, and the Cartesian materialist view of scientific objectivity to which it gives rise, are the consequence of concentrating only on the *cognitive* relation to the world. Knowing something is having a true view of it, and what is true is so independently of its being known by anyone. Truth, knowledge, have to be discovered. If someone comes to know, for instance, that Africa covers a vastly larger land area than Europe, that implies that this was true before they knew it, indeed before anyone knew it, and would have been true even if no one had ever discovered it. So in that sense, as knowing subjects we are detached from the world we know about. Descartes arrived at his conclusions about the subject of thought, as we saw earlier, as part of his attempt to lay a solid foundation for knowledge: so his conception of subject and object as separate from each other was an inevitable consequence.

But, as was argued earlier, this detached, representational relation to objects only makes objective knowledge seem difficult to account for: it leads either to scepticism or idealism. In order to know anything about the world, we must surely be *in* the world first; and the cognitive relation to objects cannot be our primary relationship to them, since it presupposes other kinds of relationship, relations of active and emotional engagement with things. My desk becomes an object of knowledge only because it was already an object for me, as something which I use in a certain way, and which has certain emotionally charged associations in my memory. These active and emotionally charged relations to the world are what some philosophers, including Merleau-Ponty, as we shall see, would call 'dialectical': there is a kind of conversation or dialectic between subject and object. In a conversation between two speakers, A and B, there is a mutual influence between what A says and what B says: what A says influences what B says in reply (it is a reply to what A has said), which in turn influences what A says in reply to that.

In somewhat the same way, the meaning which a subject finds in an object depends on how that subject regards that object, but how that subject regards the object depends on the qualities of the object. The meaning which one subject finds in an object is essentially shared with other subjects: this is most obviously so when the meaning can be expressed in words in a common language. To take a simple example, I regard the object I am sitting on as a chair (that is its meaning for me), but I can only find that meaning in it because it has the qualities required to be a chair – it has the shape, size and structure to support my weight when I sit on it. Furthermore, the meaning of the word 'chair' is part of a language shared with other subjects, the object has the meaning chair because this is how it can be used by others as well as me, so this is not just a meaning for me, but for us. Meanings don't exist in the mind, or in the object, but, as it were, in the interaction between people and objects, and between one person and others. This shows how we can avoid psychologism without postulating some kind of impersonal transcendental ego. Meanings are to be found, not by looking inside our own heads, but by investigating what we share with each other, in our common practical engagement with the world.

All this, I would argue, is contained in Heidegger's claim that the mode of being of human beings is being-in-the-world. Subjectivity, or mind, is not something detached from the world, but part of the world, interacting with objects rather than simply contemplating them. Our everyday being-in-the-world, Heidegger says, consists in our 'dealings' with the world and the entities in it; and this dealing is 'not a bare perceptual cognition, but rather the kind of concern which manipulates things and puts them to use' (Heidegger 1962: 95). Mind is thus not the name of some 'thing' which is inside us, but a way of referring to certain kinds of relationships which we can have with objects: in a sense, therefore, it is *outside* us, expressed in the ways of interacting which we share with other subjects. At the same time, as subjects, we are in the world in a different sense from that in which objects are: it is more like the sense in which someone is in a relationship with someone else. We interact with objects, which implies that the objects have an existence independent of us, and we of them, and being subjects as well as objects means, as Heidegger says, that the nature of our existence is constantly in question. We are not made what we are by the causal influence of other things, but have to ask ourselves why we should act in one way rather than another. Our very involvement with the world, paradoxically, requires us to be able to disengage from it to some extent: our minds are, as it were, semi-detached in this sense (but *only* semi).

The Cartesian idea of a totally objective world, which has so inspired the development of modern science – a world which is what it is quite apart from how we think about it, and to which our thoughts must conform – is, on this view, a myth, although it is one which has some point in some contexts. Scientists are themselves human beings, who view the world from their own perspective, limited by time and space and by their own human and individual modes of seeing. Science is one human activity alongside others: an important way of dealing with the world, but not the only one, or even the most fundamental one. It is necessary, in order to carry on with this activity, to construct an ideal view of things as they would present themselves if we could only transcend our individual, social and species limitations – a 'God's eye view', as is has been called, or what Bernard Williams called the 'absolute conception' (Williams 1978). The effort to advance in scientific understanding can then be seen as the attempt to gain such transcendence by progressively overcoming one limitation after another, but this ideal view has meaning for us only because we start from a limited view, a view from where we are, in our ordinary human dealings with the world. The scientific ideal cannot replace that limited view, or claim to be more fundamental than it: indeed, even to understand it requires us to go back to direct, concrete experience. In recognizing this, we can see a new and somewhat different role for phenomenology, which will be explored in more detail later: not as the project of seeking absolute foundations for knowledge, but as that of returning to concrete experience and refusing to substitute the abstractions of science for it.

The later Husserl and Merleau-Ponty

Scholars and commentators dispute about the extent of the influence which Heidegger's work and reputation had on Husserl, but one thing at least is clear: that Husserl's writings towards the end of his life (some not published until after his death) have a rather different tone from those of his earlier period, and reveal ways of thinking which have similarities to those of Heidegger in *Being and Time*. The terminology in many respects remains the same as that used in the earlier writings, but it is often given a different sense. There is, for example, still talk of reduction, but it is now in a different context. A central concept of the later work is that of the 'pre-given life-world' – the world in which we all, including philosophers and scientists, have our existence. In this world, we are 'objects', in the sense that we are in some particular place, alongside other objects. But we are also 'subjects', who experience the world in various ways, and from whose experience objects gain meaning or validity. We experience ourselves both as part of the world and as a point of view upon the world. Among the meanings which objects have for us are those characteristic of science – the concepts in which a scientific view of the world, or the view of things characteristic of a particular science, is expressed. But these concepts, like all the others we use in different fields, are the expressions of a particular kind of human interest in things, a theoretical interest in giving a certain kind of explanation of how things are. Part of the motivation for the later Husserl's thinking was the sense that modern European culture was in a state of crisis because of the over-emphasis on this theoretical perspective of science as the only guide to what is true and rational. This is expressed, for example, in the title of his last major work, *The Crisis of European Sciences and Transcendental Phenomenology* (Husserl 1970).

This is particularly relevant in relation to concepts of the human body. There are, Husserl points out, two distinctive ways of thinking about bodies: as what he calls the 'physical body' (for which he uses the German term *Körper*) and the 'living body' (in German *Leib*). The living body is the body as we actually experience it, primarily in our own case, as we experience our own activity and movements; the physical body is the body as thought about in science, as one object amongst others. As physiologists or doctors, for instance, we think of bodies in a detached way, in much the way that Descartes did (or a more sophisticated version of the Cartesian view). The physical body in this sense is a very complex piece of machinery whose workings are to be understood in terms of the laws of physics and chemistry. The living body, on the other hand, is not experienced from the outside in this way. For instance, the movements of my fingers in typing these words are not experienced by me as the movements of bits of matter through space, but as part of my activity in writing this book. To understand them as such is not to see them as the last stage in a causal sequence which originated in my brain and was transmitted to the fingers by electrochemical messages sent along the axons, dendrites and synapses of my nervous system. Rather, it is to grasp the reasons why I decided to write the book, and to include this chapter in it, and to choose one word or phrase rather than another in this sentence.

The living body is thus part of the life-world, the world of ordinary experience, before we begin to theorize. The physical body, on the other hand, belongs to what we may call the scientific world, the world, not of experience, but of abstract intellectual construction for the purposes of scientific theory. The phenomenological reduction, in its later version, is the business of stripping away the abstractions of science in order to get back to the life-world, which alone gives meaning to those abstractions. In the case of the body, that means seeing the experienced body, and our ways of understanding it, as primary, and the physical body, and scientific ways of understanding it, as a derivative from this primary experience, and so not deeper than it. Our neurophysiological way of understanding the movements of my fingers, for instance, perfectly valid as it is in its proper context, is not the way to understand why I am writing these words now.

This distinction between the living and the physical body provides a link between the later Husserl and Merleau-Ponty. Merleau-Ponty had been introduced to Husserl's earlier phenomenology as an undergraduate student at the École Normale Supèrieure, but does not seem to have been particularly impressed by it. What really excited him was reading an article about the later work in 1938: this inspired him so much that he went to the newly established Husserl Archive at the University of Louvain (now Leuven) in Belgium to study the texts kept there, many of which had not yet been published. The aspects of Husserl's later thought which are particularly relevant to understanding Merleau-Ponty's own philosophy, especially in relation to the themes of this book, are his conception of the life-world as the source of all meaning, his distinction between the physical body and the living body, and his (life-long) emphasis on intentionality as the mark of the subjective or mental. Merleau-Ponty also accepted Heidegger's account of human being as being-in-the-world, and the conception of the point of phenomenology which followed from it. But Merleau-Ponty, as I hope to show, developed all these themes in his own distinctive way.

Phenomenology, as developed by Heidegger, is not so much a rigorous science, seeking to uncover the absolute foundations of first-order knowledge, as an attitude of mind: it is not another theory, but a method of thinking about theories and their role in our lives as human beings. Merleau-Ponty sees this as implicit in the idea that phenomenology is concerned with *describing*, rather than *explaining*. We develop theories in order to explain our experience of the world: but that presupposes that we have an experience to be explained – experience comes before theory. In order to understand the explanatory theories, we need to go back to that starting point, and to describe what we actually experience before we begin to theorize about it. That does indeed require, as Husserl had insisted, a phenomenological reduction, a setting aside of presuppositions derived from theories in order to let our own pre-theoretical experience reveal itself. But, as mentioned earlier, that reduction can never, in Merleau-Ponty's view, be complete: absolute freedom from presuppositions is impossible, since to describe experience is necessarily to use concepts of some kind, and hence to presuppose a basic structure in what is described. The furthest we can go is to set aside the more rarefied abstractions of science in favour of those life-world concepts without which we would not have anything that could be called an experience at all.

Essentially, what this means is 'a foreswearing of science' (Merleau-Ponty 2002: ix). To foreswear science does not mean, as I interpret Merleau-Ponty, to reject scientific accounts or to deny their value. It is rather to see the limitations of science – that science cannot give a complete account of experience, because it is concerned only with the objects of experience, and leaves out of its account the subject. Scientists, as said earlier, are themselves human beings, who put forward their theories in an attempt to make sense of how the world looks from their point of view as subjects. Just as the eye by which we see things is not itself something seen, so the subject which experiences is not one of the objects which is experienced. This applies equally to the totality of subjects of experience: as subjects, they are not at the same time part of the world of objects. Science by its nature sees human beings, including scientists themselves, as a particular kind of object alongside other kinds: as living beings who are members of the species *homo sapiens*, and whose bodies function in the same way as those of other biological organisms, in accordance ultimately with physicochemical laws. The human mind or consciousness, too, is seen as an object, whose causal relationships to states and movements of the body it is one of the tasks of science to work out. However, important though these concepts of our humanity are in many respects, they cannot claim to account for the whole of reality as we experience it, because they leave out of account ourselves as subjects of experience. 'I cannot', Merleau-Ponty says, 'conceive myself as nothing but a bit of the world, a mere object of biological, psychological or sociological investigation', since these sciences themselves are sets of meaningless symbols without the subjective experience which alone gives them meaning (Merleau-Ponty 2002: ix). Phenomenology, as Merleau-Ponty sees it, might be described as a battle against what he calls 'objectivism' – simply stated, the tendency in modern culture to accept the scientific account of things as the complete truth, and as excluding what we know from our pre-theoretical engagement with the world. In some radio talks, Merleau-Ponty says:

> the question is whether science does or ever could present us with a picture of the world which is complete, self-sufficient and somehow closed in upon itself, such that there could no longer be any meaningful questions outside this picture.
>
> (Merleau-Ponty 2002: 43)

'Heidegger's "being-in-the-world"', Merleau-Ponty says, 'appears only against the background of the phenomenological reduction' (Merleau-Ponty 2002: xvi). As soon as we set aside the scientific conception of human beings as a type of object, and attempt to describe ourselves and other human beings, and the world which we experience, as we actually experience them before we construct scientific theories to explain them, we can see that human being is being-in-the-world. We are experiencers of the world, which means both that we are subjects of experience and that we are in the world in the way that objects are. But we also see that being in the world in the way that objects are entails that human beings are embodied creatures, not disembodied minds in the way that Descartes had argued. For being an object implies having a position in space, and standing in causal relations to other objects – both in the sense of affecting them and in that of being affected by them. We experience ourselves as living bodies, moving about the world and interacting with objects, but we experience our interactions with the world as more than passive responses to external stimuli: we are *agents*, active subjects, whose interactions with things can be understood in terms of the meaning which those things have for us. To reuse an already used example, my present inter-actions with my computer can be understood in terms of how I see the computer – as a word processor which I can use to write my book. Merleau-Ponty thus argues that, if we forget objectivist assumptions and attempt simply to describe how we actually experience ourselves, we will conceive of ourselves as what has been called 'body-subjects': beings who are both living organisms and experiencing subjects, and whose embodiment is inseparable from their subjectivity and vice versa. (Merleau-Ponty himself, it should be said, does not appear to use this term, but it is so commonly used by commen-tators to express his view that it may as well be used for convenience here.)

By the body referred to here must be meant Husserl's living body, rather than his physical body. For it is a *subject's* body, the body as experienced by a subject as part of him- or herself, not the body as an object, to be studied by anatomists or physiologists. I experience my own body as my presence in the world, as my point of view on the world, and at the same time as the vehicle of my actions on the world – my feet, for instance, are experienced as my possibilities of walking, my eyes as my possibilities of seeing, and my brain as my possibilities of thinking. At the same time, the nature of my body sets limits to my possibilities of experience and action in obvious ways. If I did not have feet of a particular kind, I could not walk; if I did not have eyes of the human type, I could not see the world in colour; if I did not have a brain of the kind I have, I could not think about philosophy; and so on. Saying that human beings are body-subjects is, in one way, saying that they are essentially biological creatures. But that could be misleading: they are embodied, and so biological creatures, but they are a special kind of biological creature which 'lives' their own body; or, to put it differently, which expresses, and can only express, its subjective or mental life in the movements of a biological organism.

A subjectivity which is essentially embodied is not necessarily conscious, in the sense that its experience can be explicitly articulated in words. We need to live in the world before we can give verbal expression to our experience, so that unconscious (in the sense of unarticulated) subjective experience must be at least possible. If so, then intentionality cannot be a feature only of explicit consciousness. Being afraid *of* the dark, for example, need not mean being able explicitly to identify the dark as the object of one's fear. Someone could be afraid of the dark without being able to answer the question 'What are you afraid of?', or without being able to answer it correctly (they might say, perhaps, 'I'm afraid of being burgled'). What in that case would enable us to say what the intentional object of their fear was? The most plausible answer seems to be that the intentional object is identified by seeing what best enables us to understand their behaviour. It would become clear (to themselves as well as to others) that what they were afraid of was the dark, not the possibility of being burgled, if, for instance, they did not behave fearfully in well-lit rooms, even if there was a strong possibility of burglary, and showed fear in darkened places, even when they had a police guard patrolling constantly outside. Intentionality, as this makes clear, is a feature of the person as a whole, the whole embodied subject: *I* am afraid of the dark, not my explicit consciousness or Cartesian 'mind'. My fear of the dark is not simply (and not necessarily) a matter of my having the thought of being afraid, but of a relationship in which I stand towards dark places, and which is expressed as much in my bodily reactions and behaviour as in any explicit thoughts I may or may not have.

To say that people have minds, then, is on this view not simply to say that they have explicit consciousness. It sounds plausible to say that my conscious thoughts are events or processes going on in some sense inside me, where I have guaranteed access to them and I alone have any kind of direct access to them. But if mental phenomena are not necessarily conscious, and if they are expressed in the movements of my body as much as in my articulate speech, then it sounds much less plausible to identify my mind as something inside me. To talk about my mind is, it seems, rather to talk about certain aspects of my way of being-in-the-world, of relating to things and people around me. A minimal characterization of these aspects would be that they are those which cannot be explained causally as simple responses to external stimuli, but which need to be understood in terms of the meaning which objects have for me. But this is only a minimal characterization, which needs fuller articulation in what follows. At least, however, we have now laid the basic groundwork of a conception of the mental which can provide a more adequate account of mental disorder.

Chapter 5

The body-subject and mental disorder

Human beings

To think of human beings as 'body-subjects' is to treat them, not as minds loosely attached to biological organisms, nor simply as biological organisms, but to affirm, in Ryle's words, that they are human beings. 'Human beings are human beings' is, of course, a tautology: but, like many tautologies, it makes a valuable point. In this case, the point is that we should start, in our thinking about human beings, not from some philosophical or scientific analysis, but from our actual experience of our fellows – the experience which the philosophical or scientific analysis is meant to elucidate or explain. In other words, we should approach them *phenomenologically*.

Phenomenology, at least as Merleau-Ponty understands it, is an anti-philosophical philosophy. The philosophy which it is 'anti' is that kind of traditional metaphysics which saw itself as the queen of the sciences, offering the same kind of explanation as the sciences, but at a much more profound and fundamental level. There is a certain kind of view which claims for itself the prestige of science which is, in fact, philosophical in that sense. When, for instance, people say things like, 'Science has shown that human beings are nothing but bits of living machinery', they are speaking, not as scientists, but as metaphysicians. The 'nothing but' is what gives the game away. Empirical evidence can certainly show that human beings are bits of living machinery, and that is certainly a very fruitful way of looking at some human characteristics and behaviour for some purposes. But it could not show that they were nothing but machines: that is a philosophical, not a scientific, claim. It says that this is a *complete* description of what people are: but this cannot be so, since people are also beings who, among other things, collect and evaluate empirical evidence, which entails that we need concepts in explaining and describing their behaviour which are not part of the vocabulary of mechanics – like the concepts of collecting and evaluating evidence.

The phenomenological account of human beings must be prior to any scientific or other theoretical account. A science which aims to explain the behaviour of human beings must start from the concept of a 'human being' which we all have before we even begin to do science. Otherwise, whatever it is that the science is explaining, it will not be human beings and their behaviour. We form our pre-theoretical conceptions of what a human being is from our actual encounters with other people. The other people whom we meet are certainly living beings, biological organisms, members of the same species as ourselves, but they are not only, or even primarily, that. We could not begin by thinking of them in this way, as animals who happen to belong to the same species as we do. Our interest in scientific taxonomy comes, if it comes at all, at a much later stage, and for certain specific purposes. The people we meet are, in the first instance, just *people*, beings with whom we can interact socially, as friends, enemies, strangers, passers-by, colleagues, competitors and so on.

All these forms of social interaction may well involve talking with them, but it would be misleading to concentrate too much on talking. For one thing, our social interactions go well beyond talking to others: getting on a bus, for instance, is a social interaction with the people who run the bus service, and, even if we exchange words with the driver, that is not all that social interaction consists in, or even its central element. Communication itself, furthermore, is not entirely verbal. Some people we meet are incapable of talking, or anyway of carrying on a conversation: they may have physical disabilities of one kind or another, or they may be small children who have not yet learned to talk, or people who speak a language, but not one that we understand. We can still communicate with them by non-verbal means – facial expressions, gestures, a simple touch, even sometimes that strange kind of telepathy by which we share feelings without putting them into words. Even when we do talk, our conversations are not for the most part very high-flown or intellectual: they are more likely to be such things as exchanges of everyday pleasantries (or abuse) or expressions of feeling. And there are, of course, human beings who no longer exist, or who live too far away from us to speak with us (even by telephone): we can communicate with spatially distant people by means of writing, or (in the case of the dead) they can communicate with us by means of the relics of themselves and their lives they have left, though we cannot reciprocate.

Social interactions of any of these kinds involve understanding: and what we understand is for the most part some kind of bodily expression. In speech, obviously, we need to understand the sounds uttered by the vocal chords as meaningful utterances; in writing, the marks inscribed on a page. Gestures and facial expressions are configurations of the body which have some meaning: as a smile is a certain arrangement of the face which expresses happiness, or amusement, or friendliness. But non-communicative social interactions also require us to understand what we and others are doing, and the context in which actions of this sort are appropriate. Getting on a bus, for instance, involves understanding what a *bus* is, and what it means to get on board one, and what one has to do if one is to travel by bus (such as paying the appropriate fare).

We can understand people's words and actions for the most part because and to the extent that they conform to certain norms of interpretation, which we share with them. The words which they utter or write belong to a language which we also understand and whose semantic rules give them meaning. As English-speakers, for instance, we know what is meant by the words 'Nice day today', but we also understand, in virtue of a different sort of norm, that in most contexts the point of uttering these words is not to give a meteorological commentary on the state of the weather, but as a social pleasantry, a conventional greeting. Gestures and facial expressions are subject to similar norms. A particular configuration of the face is instantly understood as a smile, and, according to the context, interpreted either as expressing benevolence, or amusement, or happiness. The smile seems to be understood in the same way by all human beings, regardless of their culture, but other gestures and expressions are understood differently in different cultures – for example, nodding the head is not always understood in the way our culture understands it, as an expression of affirmation. The understanding of actions seems to vary even more from culture to culture. Playing cricket, for instance, is liable to be seen, not as a tightly structured activity, but as a meaningless ritual, in countries which have no acquaintance with the game.

A phenomenological conception of human beings is thus not primarily as biological organisms of a given species, but as beings with whom we can have meaningful social interactions. It is not unimportant that the beings with whom we have these social interactions are members of the same biological species as ourselves, since what we understand is the bodily expressions of their thoughts, feelings, intentions, and so on, and our ability to understand them seems clearly to be conditional on our having bodies of the same structure as them. But in ordinary, non-scientific dealings with members of our own species, the bodily expressions are seen as just that – as *expressions* of thought, feeling, intention, etc. Asked to describe someone's face, for instance, we should say it was smiling, or tearful, or grimly determined, and so on, not that the bits were arranged in certain ways, or that drops of water were emerging from the eyes and trickling down the cheeks. It is impossible to smile or to cry without having appropriate biological machinery, but a person's body is not, in most everyday contexts, experienced as a piece of biological machinery. What we see is the persons themselves, expressing what they think, or feel, or intend by means of their bodies and how they work. Similarly, to explain what is going on in their bodies is not, in these cases, to describe the biological mechanisms by which the relevant bodily configurations are produced, but to say what thought, feeling, intention or whatever the person is expressing. 'Why are you smiling?', for example, would not be appropriately answered by detailing the neurological and muscular mechanisms involved in producing this arrangement of the parts of the face, but by something like 'Because I have just remembered a very good joke that was told me yesterday'.

Bodies and minds

The people that we meet, therefore, cannot be separated into bodies and minds. Their mental lives – their thoughts, feelings, intentions, wishes, hopes, plans, and so on – do not go on in some place inside their bodies, hidden from the rest of us. Their bodies are what reveals their minds. What they think is there in what they say, what they feel is bodied forth in their words, their facial expressions, and their actions, what they intend is revealed in what they do and how they do it. But this is not behaviourism in the classical sense, even though it may seem superficially like it. Behaviourists are materialists, who see human beings as physical systems like any other: for them human behaviour is therefore just a set of physical movements, to be causally explained (ultimately) by the laws of physics and chemistry. On the conception advocated here, human behaviour consists of *meaningful actions*, to be understood by grasping their meaning. For the same reason, the account given here is to be distinguished from other forms of materialism, such as the identity theory or eliminativism, according to which thoughts, for example, are identical with brain processes. On the present account, the thought that grass is green cannot be identified with the processes which undoubtedly go on in the brain of someone thinking it, but only with what would be expressed by the statement 'Grass is green', as understood by the thinker and potentially by others to whom the thinker may communicate it.

On this view, in short, the subject of thought, feeling, intention, desire, hope etc. is neither a Cartesian 'mind', existing independently of anything material, nor a 'brain', in the sense of a piece of physical machinery, operating according to physicochemical laws, but a *person*, a human being with a body (including a brain) capable of formulating and expressing thoughts, feelings, intentions, etc. It is not my mind, or my brain, which thinks the thought, say, that questions about the medical model are philosophical in character: *I* think that. I can have that thought because, first, I have a brain capable of thinking it;

second, because I understand the words used (medical model, philosophical, and so on); and third, because I have considered other thoughts which seem to me to lead to that conclusion. I understand the words used because I speak the language which contains them, and I speak that language through participating in a linguistic community in which the words are understood by others in the same way. And the process by which I move from other thoughts to this conclusion is one which I think I can justify to others, by presenting arguments which will conform to standards which they too will recognize. In all these ways, our mental life has an inescapable social dimension which prevents any simple identification with brain processes. Meanings, and so meaningful thoughts, as was argued in an earlier chapter, exist, as it were, *between* people, not *inside* them.

This suggests a way in which we can think of mental disorder, as something different from the dysfunction of some thing or system called the mind, or indeed from dysfunction of the brain. Our thoughts, feelings, intentions, etc., we can say, are disordered when they fail to conform to the appropriate social norms, and so become unintelligible, or not readily intelligible, to others. 'Normal' thoughts are those which can readily be understood by others who share the same meaning-giving norms – whether these norms govern the meaning of words, or the appropriate context in which to say something. Sometimes, the understanding is effortless, as when someone says 'Nice day today' in an appropriate context. Others may be so idiosyncratic, or original, or profound, that understanding them takes a great deal of effort, though it is nevertheless possible, as in many thoughts expressed in poetry, or science, or philosophy. Some utterances of word-like sounds may be unintelligible because they do not express a thought at all: as when someone with brain damage babbles, producing sounds any of which individually may have meaning within a language, but which are not structured in any way which would make them vehicles for a coherent, intelligible thought.

But some utterances may be so structured, and would, in another context perhaps, constitute a statement of an intelligible thought, but not in this. The last alone would be a disordered utterance in the sense intended here. It must be admitted, however, that it is not always possible in practice, so loose are the norms of intelligibility with which we operate, to distinguish between disordered utterances in this sense and those which are simply so idiosyncratic or original as to be very difficult to understand. It is not unknown, after all, for original thinkers to be regarded as mad, but if we were to look for a reasonably uncontroversial example to illustrate this sense of disordered thought, we might perhaps cite the case of someone who says to us, in a confiding tone, that the person over there is their natural father, when we know, and would assume that the speaker knows, that there is no possibility of such a connection. We can suppose that it was clear, on other grounds, that the speaker was not joking, or using the term 'natural father' in some metaphorical sense. If we asked the speaker why she said that, her answer would fail to make it intelligible to us that she should believe her statement, if the words it contains had their normal sense. And yet it would be clear that it was a statement of what she, in some sense, really thought, not just a piece of meaningless babble. She might, for instance, draw conclusions from it (e.g. 'So he ought to look after me better than he does'), or make other sorts of connections with other statements (e.g. 'But he refuses to acknowledge me').

Similar considerations would apply to emotions, desires, intentions, actions and so on. That someone should grieve over the death of someone to whom they were very close would be intelligible to us: we expect such reactions from people in such circumstances. What is much less likely to be intelligible is the *absence* of emotion in such a case, or conversely someone's exhibiting the same intensity of emotion about something which would not, in our eyes, justify it, such as the loss of a teddy bear (in adult life). Or again, we can understand why someone should wish to keep their room reasonably clean and tidy, and even admire their tidiness: we expect most people to prefer order to chaos. But someone who takes the desire for tidiness beyond normal limits – who expends energy and time on tidying up to the neglect of other life-activities, such as cooking meals or sleeping – is regarded as unintelligibly obsessive. Or, to take a final illustration, suppose someone deliberately sets fire to their own house, and gives as their reason for acting in this way something which others would regard as unintelligible, such as 'I just like to see the flames destroying all the wickedness which has taken place there'. In the absence of anything that would help us to understand that proposed justification better, we should see that person's behaviour as disordered.

The norms of intelligibility on which we rely for normal social interaction might be called human norms, and the proposal is that we should define mental disorder as thought, or utterance, or emotions, or intentions, or behaviour, etc. which is in conflict with such human norms. It is thought etc. which seems, not just difficult, but virtually impossible, for others to understand, and so which cuts off the disordered person from ordinary social interaction. Sometimes, of course, people cut themselves off from society by their own choice. An eccentric, for example, may choose a way of life which other, 'straighter', people may find it impossible or almost impossible to understand, as when someone chooses to live rough and without regard for any of the normal standards of comfort or even hygiene. The separation from straight society which this involves is a matter of choice. Or, in a different way, someone may choose a life of crime or immorality in which they deliberately defy the normal moral and legal standards of behaviour. Here, the reasons for living like this may be perfectly intelligible. The bank robber hopes to make a lot of money without too much work, which anyone can understand; the Don Juan seeks a variety of sexual pleasure without commitment, which most males, at least, can understand. In both cases, to understand is not necessarily to approve, or even to share the attitudes in question. And the understanding may be only up to a point: for instance, we may not understand why the bank robber is not inhibited, as we more law-abiding people would be, by fear of being caught and punished.

The isolation from society in such cases comes, not from unintelligibility, but from disapproval. The eccentric or the rebel may be described as in some sense mentally disordered, but neither is 'mentally ill' in the sense I shall propose here: they do not *suffer* from their social isolation, since it is chosen, an expression of what they consciously want to do. We can speak of mental illness, I shall argue, only when the person suffers from their abnormality, either through having unwanted experiences or through simply being unable through their condition to participate in normal social life as they would otherwise want to. Part of our difficulty in thinking about mental disorder is that it is all too easy to fail to distinguish between different ways in which someone's thought, or emotions, or behaviour may deviate from the norm. Eccentric, criminal, immoral and mentally ill behaviour are all abnormal, but it does not follow that they are abnormal in the same way – for instance, that all deserve compassion. There will be further discussion of the issues which arise from this in Chapter 7, after an examination of the notion of choice in Chapter 6.

In the encounters of everyday life, I have argued, we do not distinguish people's bodies from their minds. People are just people, who express their thoughts, emotions, intentions, etc. through their bodies, and whose bodily movements are intelligible as such expressions, in the same way as the thoughts etc. which they express. If mental disorder is (roughly speaking) deviation from human norms, from the norms which make possible social interaction, then what is disordered is not some part of the human being called a mind, but the human being as a whole. We interact with other human beings as embodied subjects, that is, as persons, so that what is called mental disorder might be better called personal disorder (though that might be confused too easily with personality disorder). Mental disorder is, in this sense, a disordered way of relating to the world, in particular to the human world: a disordered way of being-in-the-world, to use Heidegger's and Merleau-Ponty's expression. It is a disorder in our lives as subjects, experiencing the world in particular ways.

Later in the chapter, I shall apply this analysis to certain typical mental disorders, by way of illustration and confirmation.

For the moment, let us return to bodily disorders (bodily diseases and illnesses). For some specialized purposes, we do need to consider human bodies separately, not as vehicles for expressing mind, but simply as one other type of object in the world: that is, objectively. In the science of human biology, above all, we are concerned, not with our human interactions with other human beings, but with constructing a theoretical explanation of how the human body works which will connect it with theories about other kinds of living bodies. Even though medical practice is itself a form of interaction with other human beings (doctors with patients), the purpose of the interaction is not that of ordinary social intercourse. It is aimed at helping with certain kinds of problems which human beings face, arising from the ways in which their bodies, as living organisms, work or rather fail to work. A bodily disorder is such a problem arising from a failure in the way in which the human organism works.

To call something a disorder is, as was argued earlier, to make a value judgement – to say that it does not conform to some norms or other. In the case of a bodily disorder, as defined in the preceding paragraph, the norms in question are, in an obvious sense, *biological*. They are the standards by which we judge that a human being, considered solely as a type of living organism, and without reference to the fact that a human being is a person, is working properly. One of these norms will obviously be concerned with the human being's length of biological life: a body is disordered if it is in a condition such that the human being's chances of survival are reduced. (This is deliberately expressed somewhat vaguely. In some cases, it might mean survival until an age that would generally be considered reasonable, in others, until the age to which the human being themself might have expected to survive if they had not suffered from this condition). Another kind of norm which might be relevant has to do with the *quality* of the human being's biological life: with their ability to lead the kind of life, to perform the kinds of activities, with the degree of efficiency and energy, which anyone of their age who is considered normal can perform. A third kind of norm might concern the amount and intensity of physical pain and discomfort which a human being suffers as a result of the condition. A certain amount of pain and discomfort is an inevitable accompaniment of human, or other animal, life: it is deviation from that norm which is one criterion of disorder. A person is ill when they deviate from one or more of these norms as a result of a condition which is not chosen: thus, a love of taking risks when climbing mountains, or a preference for eating fatty foods, are not illnesses, even though they are likely to reduce the chances of survival. An organ or system of the body is diseased when it is in a state which is likely to reduce the chances of survival and/or of a reasonable quality of life, and/or to increase the level of pain or discomfort of the human being in question.

A rough-and-ready distinction can now be made between mental and bodily disorders. Mental disorders are disorders in the person's being-in-the-world, in the sense of deviations from what I have called human norms. To deviate from a human norm is to think, feel, intend, act, and so on, in ways which are not found to be readily intelligible by those considered to be normal, and so to find it impossible, or at the least very difficult, to engage in normal social interactions with other human beings. A mental disorder is one which, in this sense, affects the whole of one's being. A bodily disorder, on the other hand, consists in deviation from biological norms, as roughly defined in the preceding paragraph. It affects, not one's whole being, but only oneself considered simply as a biological organism. If I suffer from a bodily disorder, it is not *I* who am disordered, but my body: it is not working with proper biological efficiency so as to maintain the length and quality of my biological life, to spare me unnecessary physical pain and discomfort. In that sense, a bodily disorder, unlike a mental disorder, can be regarded as something which is to some degree external to the person.

This distinction, however, is very rough-and-ready, even though it may have some utility to it. The account of human beings as embodied subjects implies as much. For our being-in-the-world cannot really be separated, except in abstract thought, from our embodiment. We are, on this view, essentially biological beings: our personhood, our manner of being-in-the-world, is rooted in our biological character. We think, feel, desire, intend and act as we do because we are human beings, members of a particular biological species with particular biological structures and needs. For example, our basic desires, for food, sex, sleep and so on, and our basic emotions, of fear, anger, parental and sexual love, and the like, are those of an animal of a certain type. In a more complex culture, we also have more sophisticated desires and emotions: but the culture which gives rise to them is a developed construction out of ways of communal living which were made possible only by the bonds created by the less sophisticated biological urges and feelings. One reason, and arguably the most important one, why we can understand each other's feelings and desires is that we are members of the same biological species, who function in the same way. Personhood thus reflects biology: but conversely, as argued earlier, our biological workings are, in part at least, those of persons: the ways in which we pursue even our animal desires, or express even our basic emotions, are conditioned by the human and social context in which we pursue them.

Hence, many of the disorders we would normally classify as bodily are at least as much distorting factors in our being-in-the-world as conditions undermining our purely biological efficiency. Facial disfigurement, for instance, would be thought of as a bodily disorder, but it does not directly shorten biological life or reduce its quality. The main suffering which it causes is through its effect on our social interactions: in this respect, it could be considered as a mental disorder by the above definition. If it is thought of as a bodily disorder, this seems to be largely because it has bodily causes, and so can be most effectively treated by addressing those causes, that is, by bodily medicine. But the pain, lassitude, inability to concentrate, etc., which are the marks of bodily illness clearly have a bearing on our being-in-the-world. A converse case would be that of dementia, normally classified as a psychiatric condition, because the suffering which it results in derives from its effect on our social interactions: loss of memory disrupts our sense of personal identity, on which our social relations depend; and also undermines our capacity to recognize significant others, and to retain basic social skills. But dementia is like a bodily illness in that its causes are clearly bodily – deterioration in brain functioning – and so a treatment for it, if one were available, would be equally a part of bodily medicine – neurological repair, whether by surgery or by chemical means. So-called psychosomatic conditions, in which people suffer the symptoms of bodily illness without their usual bodily causes, and apparently for psychological reasons, are a third case in which the usual line between mental and bodily disorder becomes blurred.

What examples like these illustrate is the diversity of ways of distinguishing mental from bodily disorder, and the consequent possibility of drawing the dividing line at different points. (This is one reason why the arguments about the applicability of the medical model to psychiatry appear so difficult to resolve). In this work, however, I shall stick to the way of making the distinction which has been set out in this chapter. I believe it to draw the line at the most intuitively plausible point, such that all the paradigm cases of both mental and bodily disorder fall on the 'right' side of the division. But, as we shall see, this creates further problems about the explanation and treatment of mental disorder, which are relevant to whether such disorders are illnesses or not, as well as to a number of other issues to be considered in later chapters.

A further question which arises at this stage concerns the objectivity of concepts of health, illness and disease. Boorse's views on this question were discussed in an earlier chapter. He claimed that disease, though not illness, was an objective concept, worthy to be part of the conceptual structure of a scientific medicine: disease, for him, was a biological dysfunction, definable in entirely value-free terms. His sceptical reservations about the idea that mental disorder was an illness in the medical sense derived largely from his suspicion that such disorders cannot be equated with biological dysfunctions in the required sense. But this, I argued earlier, is confused. It is not concepts, but their use, which is evaluative or not: all concepts are defined factually, whether or not the characteristics by which they are defined are evaluated. We can, for instance, define murder as the wilful and unjustified taking of a human being's life, a factual definition on which all users of the term can agree. But murder is only used evaluatively: we do not call an act of killing murder unless we disapprove of it (that is, unless we think the killing cannot be justified). In the same way, even if (bodily) disease can be defined in terms of biological dysfunction, and biological dysfunction in terms of scientifically determinable requirements for survival and reproduction, it does not follow that disease is therefore a value-free concept. We pick out certain conditions as diseased or dysfunctional only because we value survival and reproduction, and so what is conducive to them. Evaluation, as Fulford points out, is inseparable from the way in which terms like illness or disease are used.

Nor does this in any way affect the objectivity or otherwise of the concepts in question. Boorse is still in thrall to the positivist conflation of the objective/subjective distinction with that between the factual and the evaluative: but that is itself a product of the Cartesian dualism which has such a grip on modern culture. According to Cartesian dualism, the world of objects, which science considers, is free of value or meaning, and value or meaning are merely imposed on that world from the outside by ourselves as subjects. Once we reject that dualism, however, we are free to ask whether this is really the way to think of objectivity and subjectivity. Is not the objective that which any subject can accept, regardless of his or her own subjective perspective: what is revealed by the view from anywhere, as it were, rather than the view from nowhere? On this view, the objective is more or less equivalent to the universal. By this criterion, biological norms are indeed objective: people of different cultural and individual backgrounds would agree in regarding staying alive, functioning normally, and being free of excessive pain as good things, and so would agree that what is necessary to achieve these good things is itself good. Human norms, on the other hand, seem to be much more culture-bound, and so in this sense subjective: but within a culture, there would be broad agreement on at least some human norms, since what constitutes a culture is in large part agreement on what counts as reasonable behaviour and beliefs. In any event, saying that something is a norm, whether biological or human, is expressing a value judgement. What makes modern bodily medicine scientific is not that it is value free, but that its methods of achieving its values are based on scientific knowledge. Whether the treatment of mental disorders can be regarded as part of scientific medicine in the same way depends on other considerations, to be discussed in the next section.

Causes, reasons, and illness

A minimal definition of being ill would be that it means being in an undesirable state. But, as we normally use the term, we reserve it for those undesirable states to which we are subject against our will, through the action on us of external causes: something which we therefore *suffer*. Someone who becomes extremely fat because of her love for cream cakes and her dislike of exercise, and in full knowledge of the consequences of these desires and aversions, is not 'ill' in this sense: she has chosen her condition. She may require medical treatment for the consequences of her obesity – heart problems or diabetes caused by it, for example, but her obesity itself is not an illness. (Her addiction to cream cakes and aversion to exercise might be seen by some as a *mental* illness: but to pursue that further would be a distraction at this point.)

On the other hand, obesity resulting from some biochemical imbalance in the body would be seen as an illness, because it is caused by something outside one's own control. Because its causes are outside one's own control, it is impossible to achieve a more desirable state (in this case, to cease to be obese) by an act of one's own will. Achieving that state, if it is possible at all, requires one to seek professional help of a relevant kind. The professional help is provided by someone who understands the general causes of that kind of condition, and so can identify the cause in this particular case and take the right steps to remove it. The concept of illness is thus closely connected with the idea of help based on a knowledge of causes. In this sense, to be ill is to be in a state which cannot by explained by the choice of the person concerned, but only in some other way independent of the person's choice.

Thus, whether a disorder is to be counted as an illness has a lot to do with how it is explained. Bodily illness meets that criterion because it can be explained *causally*: there is something in the body or in the external environment which causes the deviation from biological norms which we call illness. For instance, AIDS is caused by the human immunodeficiency virus attacking the body's immune system, thus rendering the body more liable to various kinds of infection. Liver disease may be caused by excessive intake of alcohol. Cancer may be caused by the effects of carcinogenic substances on the relevant bodily system. And so on. If the condition is caused by something external to the person, and so beyond her control, then it is clearly not chosen by her: she suffers it, and so it is an illness.

If this is right, then whether at least some mental disorders can also qualify as illnesses depends on whether they too can be explained in some way independent of the choice of the disordered person. Can mental disorders be explained causally, in the way that bodily disorders can? If so, then there is no problem. But to answer that, we need to discuss in more detail the nature of causal explanation. In ordinary usage, of course, the concept of 'cause' and that of 'explanation' are more or less synonymous. 'What caused that?' and 'What is the explanation of that?' mean much the same. But philosophers have traditionally attempted to give a more precise sense to cause, such that causal explanation is not a mere pleonasm, and non-causal ways of explaining something are at least conceivable. To explain something is essentially to make sense of it in some way, by answering certain kinds of question about it. But the kinds of questions which we seek to answer when we want to explain something may be different.

Sometimes, the question may be, roughly, how did that thing come about? If we discover a broken window in our house, for example, we probably want to know how it came to be broken. If we find out that it got broken when boys were playing cricket nearby and one of them hit the hard ball in such a way as to hit the window, we have our explanation. This would be a case in which it was natural to use the word cause: the cause of the window's breaking was the impact of the cricket ball on it. In identifying that as the cause of the break we are making use of our knowledge of certain generalizations: such as that the impact of hard objects like cricket balls on glass of this type normally results in the glass breaking. Similarly, if we want to know how it came about that Charles developed lung cancer while his brother James did not, and then discover that Charles was a heavy smoker while James did not smoke at all, then we may think we have answered our question: we know there is a general correlation between heavy smoking and lung cancer. This kind of explanation is connected with predictability. If we can explain the window breaking, or Charles's lung cancer, after the event, then we could have predicted them beforehand on the basis of the same evidence. If events of type A are regularly correlated with events of type B, then this enables us either to explain or to predict B, given A. A causal explanation, as it has sometimes been put, makes sense of something by showing that it was predictable in the circumstances and given our knowledge of the relevant causal generalization(s).

But we need to distinguish between mere correlations and genuine causal generalizations (causal laws). A may be regularly followed by B – so regularly, indeed, that we can reliably predict B when we see A, but it does not follow that A causes B – the correlation may be a matter of pure chance, or it may be that something else is causing both A and B. Periods of sunspot activity may be regularly correlated with periods of activity on the stock market: but it doesn't follow, and is rather unlikely, that the activity on the sun has any significant causal influence on commercial life here on Earth. In somewhat the same way, when it was first pointed out that there were statistical correlations between high use of tobacco and lung cancer, it was argued by many (not just by the tobacco companies) that this might be a mere coincidence. As these examples show, a regular correlation between events of type A and events of type B may be a necessary condition for asserting a causal relationship between A and B, but it is not sufficient. What seems to be required in addition is some intelligible linkage between A and B (something other than chance which would explain how there comes to be a correlation between the two types of event). In the case of tobacco and lung cancer, for example, it was evidence of the carcinogenic chemical effects of certain constituents of tobacco on lung tissue which seems to have been crucial.

Causal explanations, then, are the kinds we seek and need when we want to make the world or some segment of it rationally intelligible, in the sense of predictable. Technology depends on them: for it is only if we know what causes what that we are able to manipulate things to achieve human ends (which is what technology is). If we know, for instance, that heat causes ice to melt and become liquid water (that is, if we can predict that, if you heat ice, it will melt), then we can generate a water supply by gathering pieces of ice and heating them. As this example shows, this ability to predict is useful to us in our everyday practical dealings with things: heating ice to get water could be thought of either as a piece of primitive technology or as an application of common sense practical skills. In either case, we use the concept of causal explanation as a means of what might be called technological understanding of things, in which the aim is to to extract what is beneficial or avoid what is harmful in the world.

But sometimes, especially in dealing with people, and to some extent with non-human animals, we seek understanding, not for some ulterior purpose, but for its own sake. Our dealings with other human beings sometimes, it is true, benefit from our ability to predict what they will do. For example, it may be useful to an advertiser to know that consumers are likely to react in certain ways to certain kinds of visual image – that men, say, will be more likely to buy a certain make of car if it is presented as sexy, as enhancing their attractiveness to women. This kind of predictability, as in other cases, depends on knowledge of causal generalizations, in this case, to the effect that the sexual presentation of cars causes men to want to buy them. This kind of advertising is a form of technology, a way of manipulating consumer's desires. But most of the understanding on which our social relationships with each other depend is not of this technological kind. In dealing with each other in our relations in the family, in ordinary social contacts, in the workplace, in educational institutions, in trade, in courtrooms, or just as passers-by in the street, we are not for the most part seeking to manipulate each other but simply to decipher each other's actions, words, gestures and other expressions. We want to know, not how they come about (and so how we can make them come about) but what they mean, and what the person performing the action or uttering the words means by them. Making sense in this case is giving an answer to the question 'Why did she do or say that?' or 'What did she mean by that?', rather than to the question 'What brought that about?'

Most of our ordinary social dealings with each other are governed by such familiar norms that we do not need to ask the question 'Why?' or 'What do you mean?'

In reading these words, for instance, you know instantly, if you know enough English, what they mean, and from the context what I mean by writing them (I'm writing to make a certain philosophical point). We ask 'Why?' or 'What do you mean?' only in more complex or out of the ordinary cases. We see someone waving his arms on the other side of the road, and ask 'What is he doing?' (i.e. what is the meaning of his action?). We do not answer our own question by finding some generalization ('People in that situation tend to wave their arms'). Such a generalization only has a chance of being true if 'that situation' is interpreted in certain ways: it's not true, for example, if that situation means only the situation of standing at the side of a street as this man is doing. And if we can interpret the situation in such a way as to understand the connection between it and waving one's arms, we do not need the generalization. Grasping what this man means by waving his arms is not dependent on the truth of the generalization – quite the reverse. And what this man means by waving his arms in this situation is not necessarily the same as what someone else might mean by this behaviour, or what he himself means by it in other situations. Waving one's arms may be greeting someone, or doing exercises, or trying to get rid of a persistent wasp, or performing some kind of religious ritual, or expressing ecstatic joy, or many other things.

Understanding someone's meaning in doing or saying something is not related to predicting it, at least in any ordinary sense of that word. Typically, we understand someone's meaning after they have done or said something, or at the time they are doing or saying it, not before. Indeed, we can understand what they have just done when it would have been impossible to predict their action beforehand. For instance, someone may be suddenly confronted by a certain situation, unexpected either by them or by us who observe it: a total stranger, perhaps, may suddenly swear at them in the street. They may respond to this in a variety of different ways – swearing back, looking shocked, ignoring the assault, making a witty riposte, and so on. We can understand each of these responses, but could not conceivably have predicted how they would respond beforehand, even if we had known that they were about to be sworn at.

Another way of making this point would be to say that our understanding of their response does not depend on knowledge of any generalizations about the way in which they as individuals, or people of their type (however defined), or people in general respond in such cases. There may be no such (true) generalizations, or, if there are, we may not know them. What we have instead are certain shared conceptions of what constitutes an intelligible response, given the significance (a grasp of which we also share) of swearing at someone else. In part, we share these conceptions because of our common humanity; in part, the sharing is peculiar to a particular culture which we have in common with the person we understand. And in some particularly difficult and idiosyncratic cases, we can grasp what someone means, with great difficulty, without any pre-existing shared conceptions, by using our imagination to 'put ourselves in their shoes': we might do this when trying to get the sense of a particularly obscure poem, or to understand some extremely bizarre behaviour.

It is not simply the case, as a matter of fact, that we can have this kind of understanding of the meaning of people's words and actions without being able to predict them: this kind of understanding is *conceptually* unrelated to predictability. To provide a causal explanation of something that happens is to make sense of it, as was suggested above, by seeing that it was predictable in the circumstances. But to understand the meaning of an action is to make sense of it just by grasping what kind of action it is, which is determined by what it means to the person acting, the agent. This kind of understanding is constitutive of social life. To have a social relationship of any kind with someone else is possible only to the extent that one understands that person's actions, words and other expressions. The closer the relationship, the deeper one's understanding of the actions etc. has to be. Our superficial relationships to the strangers we encounter in everyday life depend on only a minimal understanding of what they are doing: this person is serving at the till in the supermarket, this person is the driver of the bus who collects the fares, and the like. Our relationships to colleagues require a more subtle understanding, and our relationships to close friends, spouses, lovers, parents or children depend for their existence on an extremely sophisticated understanding of the meanings of the things they do, say and otherwise express. (In all these cases, of course, the understanding must be mutual if the relationship is to exist at all). In general, at all levels, understanding of meaning is essential to our coexistence as human beings: it involves regarding others *as* fellow human beings to be related to, not as objects whose behaviour is to be predicted.

The distinction which I have made between understanding the meaning of an action, word, or other expression and causal explanation has been made in different ways in the literature. Some German philosophers and social scientists of the nineteenth century and after labelled the understanding of meaning *Verstehen* (the German word for understanding) and kept *Erklären* (German for explanation) exclusively for causal explanation. One of the greatest philosophers of psychiatry, Karl Jaspers (1883–1969) follows this line in his *General Psychopathology* (Jaspers 1997), as, more recently, do Bolton and Hill (see below). But this is misleading in some ways: both are types of explanation, and both attempt to understand – they just explain/understand different things in different ways and for different purposes. Other philosophers recognize this and distinguish between reason-explanation and causal explanation. Reason-explanation corresponds to what I have called understanding of meanings, since to understand the meaning of someone's words or actions could be described as seeing their reasons for saying what they say or doing what they do. The unfortunate thing about this designation, however, is that it tends to imply that only actions performed, or words spoken, with a conscious or rational purpose in mind can be understood, whereas it seems desirable from the point of view of our present topic to include unconscious meanings and purposes and their understanding. I propose therefore to use the terms 'meaning-explanation' and 'causal explanation' from now on.

Meaning-explanation and causal explanation, as should now be clear, are distinct modes of making sense of phenomena. In giving a causal explanation of something that happens, we make sense of it by showing how it was brought about, how it was predictable given our knowledge of certain causal generalizations about the connections between types of events and of the particular surrounding circumstances on this occasion. Causal explanations can be given of any type of phenomenon, including human actions. We can give a causal explanation of my raising of my arms, for example, in terms of the processes in my brain and nervous system and in my muscles which led to this happening. This explanation would apply equally well to any other similar movement in organisms of the same kind: in other words, it is not specifically an explanation of *my* raising my arms, but of this kind of arm movement in general.

If we want to know, on the other hand, why I raised my arm at that time, we are asking, not what brought it about that my arm moved in this way, but why I raised my arm at that time – what *my purpose* in raising my arm at that time was. It might be expressed differently: what exactly was I doing when I raised my arm? The answer might be, as was said earlier, that I was waving to a friend, or trying to get rid of a wasp, or doing some exercises, or one of many other things. The explanation would be specific to this particular action, performed by me at this time: I myself, on other occasions, or other people, might well have different reasons for raising the arms. Assigning a meaning to an action, as said earlier, does not make it intelligible by indicating how it came about, or by showing that it was predictable in the circumstances: it makes the action intelligible by showing that the meaning it expresses is shared between the agent and the person who seeks to understand the action. For this reason, it can *only* be used to make sense of actions, because only what counts as an action can be said to have a meaning in the relevant sense. An action is defined as what it is by the meaning which the agent gives it, or by the reasons they have for performing it. In the example, the same movement (raising one's arms) can constitute different actions, each defined by the purpose for which it was performed.

Movements of matter through space are identified as what they are without reference to any meaning (indeed, most movements do not have any meaning). Thus, we could define the movement here as constituted by the object which moves (in this case, a human arm) and the spatial positions between which it moved (from a downward-pointing position beside my hips, say, to one in which it pointed upwards beside my head). That completely distinguishes this movement from others, and so indicates what has to be explained, in terms of causes rather than of meanings. If we take seriously the idea of human beings as body-subjects, we can see that there can be no human action without a relevant bodily movement, where relevant means 'of a type appropriate for performing that action'. I can't greet my friend by waving except by moving my arm in a particular way. This has interesting consequences for the explanation of both actions and movements. It means, first, that we can give both causal and meaning-explanations of actions in different respects: putting it differently, in different contexts we can ask both 'How did it come about?' and 'Why did he or she do it?'. The two types of explanation, though different, in a sense apply to the same thing. Causal explanation of the movements involved in performing the action, second, is a statement of the necessary conditions for the action to be possible. The repertoire of human actions can include this kind of greeting, for instance, only because human bodies are of a sort which can move in the relevant way.

Similar points can be made about thoughts, emotions, moods, desires, wishes, hopes, and so on. I can think 'There's my friend Paul, I must greet him' only because I have a brain of such a kind as to make this sort of thinking possible. I can have a desire to eat something only because the human body is so constituted as to give rise to feelings of hunger. I can feel amused at someone's joke only because my brain is of a kind which allows such feelings. In general, the kinds of meaning which human actions (including speech acts), thoughts, emotions, desires, etc. can have is limited by the nature of human beings as biological organisms, and failures in the mechanisms of the human body, including the brain, can explain why meaningful actions of certain kinds become impossible. Conversely, however, the workings of the human body as a biological organism are themselves meaningful – its movements are not purely mechanical, but have to be understood as expressions of the life of a human being. The workings of the brain, in particular, and of the cerebral hemispheres above all, have to be understood, not simply in terms of bio-logical efficiency, but also in terms of their contribution to the personal life. Unlike the heart, say, whose function is entirely to do with sustaining biological life, the functioning of the brain is at least as much to do with making possible personal life. Brain processes can, in this sense, be intentional – definable in terms of their directedness to achieving certain human goals: though it is not so much the brain process as such which is intentional as the person's action, of which the brain process forms an essential part.

Both sorts of explanation thus help to make human action intelligible. But that in itself only emphasizes that they are *different* sorts of explanation – that one kind cannot be reduced to the other. There is a standing temptation to philosophers, in particular, or philosophically minded scientists, to think that only causal explanation is really acceptable as rational or 'scientific', so that meaning-explanation either has to be rejected altogether, or has to be shown to be a peculiar kind of causal explanation. It is easy to see why this con-clusion should seem so plausible. Causal explanations certainly look more objective than meaning-explanations. The movements of my arms through space can be identified as what they are independently of whether anyone is observing them, or of the particular perspectives of particular observers, includ-ing their cultural perspectives. They are surely, we feel inclined to say, matters of fact, not opinion. The meaning of my action, on the other hand, depends very much on what I think it is, and its intelligibility to others depends on whether they think like me or not. In this sense, it is subjective. And if we follow the traditional Cartesian model, referred to already several times in this book, we shall think of the subjective and the objective as mutually excluding each other. In science, we are supposed to seek objectivity: scientific explanations must therefore be in terms of the objective notion of causality, not in terms of the subjective notion of meaning. If we further think, according to the dominant view of our culture, that science is the only paradigm of rationality, then to indulge in any form of meaning-explanation which is not a special form of causal explanation will be to descend into subjectivism and irrationality.

In their excellent book *Mind, Meaning and Mental Disorder* (Bolton and Hill 2003), Derek Bolton and Jonathan Hill give an account of meaning-explanation which is plainly influenced by this line of thinking. They rightly accept the criticism of old-style behaviourism, which attempted to explain human behaviour in mechanistic terms of 'stimulus' and 'response', that it fails to do justice to the goal-directedness and plasticity of much human behaviour, and also, for that matter, of significant portions of the behaviour of non-human animals. The purposiveness and plasticity of behaviour are expressed, in the terms used above, in the fact that the same movements may constitute different actions, and indeed that the same action may be embodied in different movements (as one may greet someone by waving, by nodding and smiling, by shouting 'Hello!' and so on). To account for purposiveness and plasticity, they say, we must allow for the subject's contribution: what makes moving one's arm in a certain way a greeting in one case and an attempt to rid oneself of a wasp in another is that this is the meaning of the action as seen by the subject in each case.

Thus far, I would have no disagreement with what they say – but it is at this point that disagreement begins. Following Chomsky's critique of Skinner's views on language, and the wider cognitive revolution in psychology, Bolton and Hill identify the subject's contribution with 'internalized structures and rules' (Bolton and Hill 2003: 8) or with 'a representation of the environment' (2003: 9). Whereas stimulus–response theories treat the information which regulates behaviour as already present in the external environment, this cognitive approach sees that work needs to be done *within* the system in processing information (2003: 11). The meaning which a human action has is thus equated with a mental state, an item within the mind: the explanation which it provides is then said to be causal – the mental state is the cause of the action in the same way that the impact of the stone on the window is the cause of its breaking. The argument used in support of the contention that meaning-explanation is in this way a form of causal explanation is that it allows actions to be predictable in just the same way as other causal explanations (Bolton and Hill 2003: 43). And this form of mentalistic causation is then linked with neurophysiological causation by saying that the meaning is 'encoded' in the brain (2003: 61).

This view, or something like it, is not found in Bolton and Hill alone, but is part of a distinguished philosophical tradition. Nevertheless, to treat reasons or meanings as a type of causes is to misunderstand the nature and purpose of meaning-explanation. It is what Merleau-Ponty criticizes, in several places, as causal thinking – effectively, thinking that only causal explanation counts. To explain an action, emotion, desire etc. by giving its reason, or its meaning for the person concerned, is not to identify a discrete antecedent event which brought about the action or whatever as its effect. It is to identify the action etc. itself as what it is. Thus, if you ask what I am doing at the moment, I might reply 'I am writing a chapter of my book'. This identifies what I am doing in tapping the keys of my word processor and staring at the screen, and distinguishes it from other actions which I might perform by making the same movements – such as playing a computer game or writing a letter to the bank. In so doing, it explains what I am doing sitting here at my desk: you know the reason why I am typing. But it does not do so by identifying a cause which brings it about that my fingers are making these movements. There is such a cause – namely, the processes in my brain, nervous system and muscles which eventuate, according to normal laws of physiology, in finger-movements of this type. But these neurological and muscular processes are not identical with my reasons for acting as I do, any more than 'moving my fingers' is identical with 'typing a chapter of my book'.

Moreover, the relation of reason to action is not an instance of an empirical generalization, which could form the basis for a rational prediction. There is no true generalization that a desire to write a book brings about movements of fingers on a keyboard, which would enable anyone to predict that if I have decided to write part of my book this afternoon, I shall be seated at my computer and my fingers will be working in this way. Writing a book can be realized, among other ways, by hand-writing, by dictating to a tape recorder, or to a secretary, even by going for a walk and thinking what one is going to say. And, as authors know only too well, the desire to write a book may be followed by no action at all, so that one cannot even predict, from the knowledge of my desire to get on with my book, that I will perform one of a finite set of movements. We do not make sense of each other's actions (words, emotions, desires, etc.), through empirical knowledge of reason–movement connections. Karl Jaspers recognized this, when he said that our conviction of understandable connections 'is not acquired inductively *through repetition of experience*' (Jaspers 1997: 303, his italics). We acquire it rather through being human ourselves, and so sharing certain conceptions of possible reasons for action. And in many cases we share it through participating in a culture in which certain types of movements normally have one of a range of possible meanings, and in which certain purposes are reasons for performing certain kinds of actions. Not empirical laws, but shared norms of intelligibility, are the basis for meaning-explanations.

Why are you sitting at your computer? I'm writing part of my book. But why are you writing your book today? Because I want to get it finished to meet the publisher's deadline. What we want to know is the point of doing something, and it would not answer our question, as was said earlier, to be told what brought it about that our bodies move in this particular way. We want to know it, furthermore, as was said above, not in order to predict what others will do, but in order simply to understand their actions as part of our living together with them. Since we are essentially embodied creatures, people can have reasons for acting, and can give meaning to their actions, only because certain things go on in their brains: but their reasons are not, and could not be, encoded in their brains, because to have a reason for doing something is more than just to have certain processes going on in one's brain.

What is this something more? It is belonging to, actively participating in, a human society in whose activities the relevant concepts get their meaning. To have a desire to write a book, for example, one must belong to a culture in which books and their writing have a particular place, in which the expression 'writing a book' has a meaning which is widely understood. Writing a philosophical book about psychiatry also involves having the concepts of philosophy, of psychiatry, and of the philosophy of psychiatry: having such concepts is possible, again, only because one has a brain capable of formulating and grasping them, but it cannot be equated with the processes going on in one's brain when exercising this capacity. One can have such concepts only if others share them, if they are part of a collective activity in which one, as a whole human being, not just a brain, engages along with others. In this sense, the reasons for acting are not, as has been said more than once already, 'in someone's head' or 'in someone's brain', but out there, in the space of ideas that one inhabits with other human beings – part of our being-in-the-world. Brains don't think: people do (and use their brains in doing so).

Does this account of meaning-explanations make them intuitive and subjective, and so remove them from the realms of science? If we are uncertain whether we have the objectively correct causal explanation of some phenomenon, we can test it in a way which any rational being could accept. That is, we can derive predictions from our proposed causal law, and see whether these predictions are confirmed by the facts. It is not a matter of opinion, but of solid fact, that heating water to 100° at sea level causes it to boil, as can be tested by trying the experiment. But if meaning-explanations do not give rise to predictions, they cannot be tested in this way. How then do we know which of the possible explanations for a particular action, statement, desire or emotion is the correct one: is it even possible to speak of a 'correct' meaning-explanation, or is it just a matter of what happens to satisfy a particular explainer? Jaspers recognizes this problem: a particular 'meaningful connection', he says, may seem 'self-evident', but it does not follow that it is 'really there' or even that it occurs in reality at all (Jaspers 1997: 303). Whether it is real (e.g. whether my desire to get on with my book is the real reason for my sitting typing now) depends, he goes on to say 'on the tangible facts (that is, on the verbal contents, cultural factors, people's acts, ways of life, and expressive gestures) in terms of which the connection is understood, and which provide the objective data' (his italics). In the example, it is as clear as anything can be, given my circumstances and other things about my life, and given the words which are actually appearing on my monitor now, that getting on with my book is the real motivation for what I am doing, and not, say, fooling around to pass the time. In other cases, Jaspers says, there is more room for divergence of interpretation, and so much less possibility of certainty: this applies particularly, according to him, in attempting to understand psychiatric patients. The inability to find a decisive interpretation of someone's behaviour which must be accepted by all rational beings does not, however, make interpretation purely subjective, in the way in which judgements of taste are. There may not be definitively correct interpretations, but there can certainly be better- and worse-supported ones, and the distinction depends on how good a case an interpreter can make, using evidence, for a particular understanding. Understanding human behaviour may not be an exact science, like physics, but it does not follow that it is therefore a mere matter of irrational or non-rational intuition.

If the central core of mental disorders are, as argued earlier in the chapter, distortions in our normal mode of being-in-the-world, then that suggests that they require a meaning-explanation as well as, or perhaps rather than, one in causal terms. If we say that a schizophrenic's way of perceiving the world is a problem for us because it is delusive, out of touch with reality, so that we cannot participate with him or her in a common human life, then what we need is to understand why he or she thinks in that way. Why does he see himself as the victim of a conspiracy, when no other people can see any evidence for this? This is at least as important a question to try to answer, if we want to help him, as 'What goes wrong in the brains of schizophrenic people with delusions of persecution?' Similarly, if a person is afraid to go out into open spaces, or refuses to eat on the grounds that she is too fat (which we can plainly see not to be the case), or believes herself to be a machine, or to be dead, or is afraid to step on the lines between paving-stones, or continuously washes her hands, the question we need to ask is 'Why?', not 'What mechanism is responsible for this behaviour?' The behaviour is not equivalent to a set of bodily movements, but to an *action*, which has a meaning for the agent: if it is disordered behaviour, that is because it does not, at least at first sight, appear to have any meaning for us, because it does not fit into any of our standard norms of intelligibility. But if it had no meaning, it would not be an action at all, whether normal or disordered. The static in a radio signal is not a disordered communication, because it is not a communication at all, just a meaningless effect of certain atmospheric causes.

This view of mental disorder as having a meaning, but just not a standardly intelligible meaning, gives rise to further questions which will be discussed in the next chapter. Does it imply that causal explanation has no role to play in the case of mental disorder? And if it does, does that rule out any conception of mental disorder as a form of (medically treatable) illness?

Chapter 6

Mental disorder and choice

Illness as suffering

Words like 'ill', 'illness' and even 'disease' are not, as was noted in an earlier chapter, precisely defined technical terms, but get their meaning from their use in ordinary discourse. Nevertheless, there are certain limits on their proper use, at least in their standard sense. Being ill is being in an undesirable state, but not any kind of undesirable state will count. It must be a state, as was argued in the last chapter, which one *suffers*: that is, one which is undesirable to the person in that state, and so which is not the result of that person's own deliberate choice. To be unconcerned about the sufferings of others, for instance, is to be in an undesirable state, but the callous person herself does not think of it as such, and has a choice (presumably) about whether to be in that state or not. So callousness is not an illness. To be unable to breathe properly because of pneumoconiosis is to be in a condition which no one would want to be in, and which no one therefore would choose to be in – pneumoconiosis thus is an illness. There are some further qualifications which need to be made to this account. First, not all suffering resulting from unchosen conditions counts as illness. Human life inevitably involves a certain amount of unavoidable pain and distress, and this 'normal suffering' is not regarded as illness: illness is essentially *abnormal* suffering. Second, we regard an undesirable condition as illness only if it is more than momentary: if I accidentally cut my finger on a knife, and feel a short-lived pain as a result, then no one would say I was ill. Given these qualifications, the crucial point about illness is that it is being in a condition which one finds undesirable and which was not the product of one's own deliberate choice. That is why we think the appropriate attitude to an ill person is sympathy, rather than condemnation; and why we have developed medicine, to help to remove or alleviate illness when the sufferers cannot do this by their own efforts.

In some cases, it might be pointed out, people do make themselves ill by their own choices. Choosing to indulge in excessive consumption of alcohol may lead to cirrhosis of the liver; choosing to smoke tobacco can lead to lung cancer, heart disease and so on. Are not these examples of illness as chosen? They certainly look like that, and in some situations it may be useful to think of them in that way – for the purposes of health promotion campaigns, for instance – but perhaps for our present purposes it is better to interpret them differently. For simplicity's sake, let us concentrate on one example, that of cirrhosis resulting from excessive drinking. In this case, it might be said, what people choose to do is to indulge in more pints of beer, or glasses of wine or whisky than is wise. Although they may know that this is likely to lead to health problems, they are not choosing to have those problems: if asked whether they wanted to run the risk of premature death as a result of their indulgence, they would almost certainly answer 'No, I just like drinking'. In this sense, it is not strictly the case that they have chosen the cirrhosis which results from it. Something can be an indirect consequence of a free choice, without itself being freely chosen. Someone whose suffering is ultimately the result of their own choice may be less deserving of sympathy, but they are nevertheless still suffering, and so ill.

All this has a clear bearing on the question of whether mental disorders are to be called illnesses. First, it plainly follows that behaviour, or thought, or affect, or desire which is disordered in the sense that it deviates from the standard human norms is not mental illness unless it results in suffering for the person concerned, in the sense of seeming undesirable to them. Eccentricity, however hard it may be for 'normal' people to understand, and however much it may interfere therefore with many normal human inter-actions, is not illness. The loner, for instance, who genuinely does not wish for company, may be regarded as crazy by the rest of society, but cannot be called mentally ill on the present account. It is even more obvious that other forms of behaviour which were at one time classified as mental illness, simply because they deviated from the conventional norms of society, were wrongly so described: homosexuality, for instance. If someone accepts their sexual orientation, then it is, in that sense, chosen, and so is not an illness: inability to accept it may be an illness, because that makes the orientation something one suffers, but that is a different story.

Second, the requirement that an illness should involve abnormal suffering means that we cannot describe any mental distress which is part of the normal human condition as part of a mental illness. As well as being full of pain, human life is full of unhappiness. No one can participate in human relation-ships without running the risk of loss, either by the death of the other person or by the break-up of the relationship. Friends, parents, children, spouses, lovers die, and human beings suffer grief as a result. This grief is unchosen, but it is not an illness: it is part of the price we must pay for emotional closeness – far from interfering with human interactions, it is a necessary part of a human interaction worthy of the name. Much the same applies to the distress we feel at unrequited love, or at the end of a marriage, an affair or a friendship. Being disappointed in one's ambitions, though distressing, is similarly a normal part of life, not an illness. Again, these situations are not even mental disorders, by the account given in the previous chapter, since they are not distortions in our mode of being-in-the-world in the sense of interfering in our normal human interactions with others, and they are readily intelligible to all normal human beings.

There is one respect in which the account of mental disorder given in the previous chapter might seem, at first sight at least, to rule out treating *any* mental disorder as mental illness. It was argued there that distortions in our mode of being-in-the-world need to be understood in terms of reasons or meanings, rather than, or as well as, being causally explained. This might seem to imply that mental disorders are chosen, and so are not forms of illness. The generally recognized bodily illnesses are, as argued there, clearly not chosen, because they are the outcome of causes, not of our free choice. They are caused by infection, or injury, or the chemical effects of substances, or by genes, on their own or in combination with environmental factors. What all these causes have in common is that they are *external* to the sufferer, not within his or her conscious control. What links causes to effects is impersonal law, not personal choice. If I am infected with the flu virus, and if my immune system does not produce antibodies to resist the invader, then I will get flu, whether I like it or not. But a meaning-explanation makes what I do intelligible in terms of the reasons which influence me, not in terms of causes operating from outside me. Why am I writing this book? Because I believe I have things to say on these topics – in other words, because it fulfils one of my own purposes. I have *chosen* to write it. In general, meaning-explanation implies choice, and choice implies meaning-explanation.

So if mental disorders require meaning-explanation, that seems to imply that they are chosen ways to behave, think, feel, desire, and so on, not illnesses which we suffer. They look more and more like the 'problems in living' which Szasz speaks about (e.g. Szasz 1972: 243). Some mental disorders may escape this objection. For instance, disorders which consist, wholly or mainly, in the loss of a mental capacity can be completely explained causally in terms of the loss or deterioration of the brain connections which are necessary to the capacity in question. Alzheimer's disease is a case in point which has already been cited: its symptoms seem to be the result of the loss of certain memory capacities due to deterioration in the brain, and so it is clearly not the outcome of choice, and can be classified as an illness – though a neurological illness. There is the complication that, because our capacities to remember and to recognize others are so central to our being-in-the-world, there is a case for regarding it also as a mental disorder. Be that as it may, however, the argument for describing it as an illness depends on the assertion that it resembles bodily illnesses in having a purely causal explanation.

In other cases, however, this argument does not seem to hold. Mental disorder may be reflected in processes in the brain, and it may indeed be the case that the disorder could not happen without such processes, but it does not follow that these brain processes causally explain the disorder, or that they explain it at all. If one accepts, as a non-dualist, that thought, emotion, desire and so on are possible only if certain parts of the brain are functioning, then one would have no mental processes at all (including those we call 'disordered') unless the brain was operating in appropriate ways. So one could not have any moods, say, whether disordered or not, unless one's brain were functioning. By the same token, the nature of brain functioning cannot explain the difference between a disordered mood and one which is not disordered – between, to use an earlier example, anxiety about venturing into open spaces when there is no real danger and the anxiety of a frail old person about venturing into the streets when there is a genuine risk of being the victim of crime. It may well be that neurological or biochemical factors can explain, in some cases, the fact that some people are more likely than others to respond to situations in ways we regard as disordered; but it is nevertheless the response itself which needs to be explained, not the propensity to it. We might draw a parallel with someone who has a genetic predisposition, say, to have high levels of cholesterol in the blood: it is not this on its own, however, which explains why they actually have high levels of cholesterol, but the nature of their dietary intake, which activates the disposition. In the same way, someone may be more prone (for whatever reason) to feel anxiety than most, but to explain why they actually feel anxiety at present we need to explain what it is in their environment that they find anxiety-provoking. In other words, we need to give a meaning-explanation. So does that mean we have to treat the anxiety as freely chosen?

Choosing

I want to argue that this appears to be a problem only because we have an unrealistic conception of what human choice involves, and of the relation between meaning-explanation and causal explanation. We have an idealized picture of choosing as a process in which we consciously and rationally examine various alternatives, weighing them against each other in the light of equally conscious values and on the basis of that weighting coming down in favour of the alternative which seems best in accord with those values. We choose a new car, let us say, on the basis of its price, its fuel efficiency, its mechanical reliability, its comfort, its looks, its suitability for our needs (e.g. the amount of space for passengers and luggage), and so on. Different people may use different criteria, or give different weightings to those mentioned. A car which we genuinely *choose* will be one which seems to us, on the basis of the information we have to hand, best to fit our criteria and our weighting of them. External factors may, however, interfere with our freedom of choice. The boss may insist, despite our protestations, that we buy a car which does not meet some of our most important criteria; or we may be forced, because of lack of money, to take a car which is less than satisfactory but is more affordable. Then we might be said to 'suffer' the car we have acquired because it was not what we should have chosen.

That this example is a case of choosing is undeniable, but the idea that this is what choice always means has force for us only because we are still in the grip of Cartesian ways of thinking. Choosing clearly involves the mind: we can be said to choose at all only because we can think, can evaluate things in terms of purposes, and thought and purpose are mental concepts. For the Cartesian, 'mind' is defined in terms of consciousness and reason: anything which is not fully conscious is thus, for Descartes, not part of the mind, but something material, part of the material world which operates in terms of mechanical causation. A choice worthy of the name must therefore, for the Cartesian, be a decision arrived at as the result of conscious thought, in which the possibilities are evaluated in the light of consciously held principles. Furthermore, these principles must be rational in character – otherwise they would not be describable as principles. An impulsive movement could not be said to be freely chosen, because it was the outcome not of thought or reflection, but of a mere impulse which, as such, must belong to the body, not the mind. Acting on the basis of a principle, however, is behaving in a way which commends itself to thought, and that must mean, which is rational. And rational principles are, as argued earlier, those which are intelligible to anyone, which conform to generally accepted standards of intelligibility. Anyone can see that fuel efficiency is desirable in a car (whether or not it is at the top of their list of criteria), and so that it is rational to choose a car on that basis, but if someone bought his car on impulse, because of feeling happy at the time, perhaps, and without regard to its manifest defects by ordinary standards, then we might, to say the least, doubt the rationality of his purchase. In Cartesian terms, we should also doubt whether it was a real choice.

There must, however, be something wrong with this model of choice – it must at the very least be an over-simplification. To choose to act in a certain way is contrasted with being *made* to act in that way. The chosen act is *one's own* action; being *made* to act is acting because of something *outside* oneself. On the Cartesian view of human beings, one's self is identical with one's mind, that conscious subject which is utterly distinct from anything else in the universe, even the human body. So it is logical for a Cartesian to give the above account of choice as conscious, rational decision-making, and as that alone. But we have seen the problems with the Cartesian view of human beings as disembodied consciousnesses, so that it is equally logical for us to question the view of choice which is derived from it.

If we do not make Cartesian assumptions, then there seems no reason, for instance, to deny that an impulsive action is as much an expression of choice as one resulting from careful thought and deliberation. My impulses are surely as much a part of me as my reflective thoughts: they are not imposed on me from outside. They are not the same kind of thing as, for example, reflexes like the knee-jerk reaction. An impulse (in the sense we are concerned with here) is intentional, whereas a reflex is not. The reflex is defined as what it is simply by its physical characteristics: it is a movement of the knee which generally happens when the knee is tapped in a certain way. An impulse, however, is defined as what it is by its directedness towards a certain intentional object: it is an impulse *to buy a car*, as opposed, say, to one *to hug a tree*. The directedness almost certainly involves some kind of thought – being happy could not make one buy a car unless one knew what a car was, and how one might buy one. These are one's own thoughts, and so the decision comes from within oneself, not from outside, but the thought is not made conscious, and it is not governed by generally accepted standards of rationality.

Other intentional states and processes can be chosen, in the sense of being one's own, rather than imposed from outside, but are responses to the world rather than actions, and need not be the result of rational, conscious deliberation. Emotions and moods, for example, are intentional: we are happy or sad *about* something, fearful *of* something, angry *at* something, and so on. Similarly with desires: we want *something* or *someone*. This directedness may involve thought: we may have come to be afraid of global warming, say, because we have thought about its dangers. But it need not be: if I see a hungry lion prowling in the jungle, I immediately and without the need for reflection feel afraid. Whether or not they are the product of conscious thought, my emotions are *my* emotions, not something imposed on me from the outside (unless they are induced in me by hypnosis – but hypnosis can only work in this way because most of the time emotions are one's own responses to things outside). I have my reasons for feeling them: hungry lions *are* dangerous. Much the same may be said about desires. I may have come to want a camcorder because I have thought about it and how it might be useful to me; but equally I can desperately want an apple when I am very hungry without the need for any kind of reflection. In either case, again, my desires are equally mine, and they equally have reasons – I want the apple because I know it will alleviate my hunger, or because it looks so juicy. In this sense, emotions and desires are as much chosen as actions. Moreover, emotions and desires, because of their intentionality, are intelligible to others, to the extent that the reasons for having them are such as to conform to generally acceptable norms of intelligibility.

The body-subject and choice

To account for this, we need a different account of minds and bodies from the Cartesian. In this book, I am advocating such an alternative account, namely, Merleau-Ponty's conception of human beings as 'body-subjects'. On this conception, as we saw, a human being is not a combination of two quite separate (though interacting) parts, a body and a mind, but a unity in which the thinking subject is necessarily embodied, and in which the lived body has to be understood as the expression of subjectivity. In simpler terms, my self (or that of any other human being) is not some kind of disembodied soul, but the human being that I see in the mirror when I shave, or who was photographed years ago playing with my children. This is a materialist con-ception in one sense, namely, that it does not propose the existence of any non-physical substance. But it is not materialist in the sense of *reducing* human beings to mere bits of matter: that is, of saying that, in the last analysis, all human properties and relations can be fully described and explained in the language of physics. When I was playing with my children, all my movements were governed by the laws of physics. But 'playing with one's children' is more than moving a lump of matter (one's body) through space from point A to point B, and then to point C. It is doing things: for instance, intentionally throwing a ball to one's child (recognized as one's child), in the hope that he will catch it. 'Intentionally throwing', 'recognizing someone as one's child', and 'hoping that he will catch it' do not belong to the vocabulary of physics, nor are they logically equivalent to any terms in that vocabulary. Physics, we might say, involves a different way of thinking about human beings and their actions, as sets of movements of matter through space: but it is not truer or more fundamental than the way of thinking which sees what I was doing as 'playing with my children'. Rather, the latter is the more fundamental, because it gets its meaning from the ordinary human experience which must precede the development of physics.

No one, of course, could play with their children in this way unless they were embodied beings: playing ball with one's children involves making some kinds of physical movements. Even playing mental chess with them involves movements in the brain, the transmission of messages between neurons. All this follows from acceptance of our essential embodiment, but the conception of ourselves as embodied *subjectivities* entails that these physical movements themselves have to be understood, not simply in terms of the laws of physics, but as necessary parts of the way in which a subject expresses themself. The body in question is not an object in the world like any other, it is *my* body, and its movements are *my* movements: they have to be understood in terms of their meaning for me – in short, as intentional. The notion of the body-subject extends the scope of subjectivity and intentionality, in short, beyond the realm of explicitly conscious thought to include the whole 'lived' body. Behaviour can be understood in terms of its meaning for the subject even if that subject has not consciously thought about its meaning.

Intentionality is a feature, on this view, not of consciousness, but of living and conscious beings. For to be a living being is to function, not merely as a collection of separate parts, but as an organism, an organized whole which interacts with its environment in a purposive way. An organism as such has needs – the most basic of which is simply to stay alive – so that its relation to its environment is not simply one of passive response to external stimuli but one of active attempts to meet those needs. Merleau-Ponty sees this way of thinking as applying even to very primitive types of organisms such as the insect which he discusses in *Phenomenology of Perception* (Merleau-Ponty 2002: 90). The insect has had one of its legs cut off: in the performance of an 'instinctive act', it substitutes a sound leg for the missing one. This, Merleau-Ponty argues, cannot be explained mechanically, as an automatic substitution of a stand-by device, since the same does not happen when the leg is merely tied, and not amputated. But neither, of course, does the insect have a conscious aim in mind. Rather, Merleau-Ponty says, 'the tied limb is not replaced by the free one, because it continues to exist in the insect's scheme of things, and because the current of activity which flows towards the world still passes through it' (loc. cit.).

The claim is, then, that the difference between the behaviour with the tied leg and that with the amputated leg can be explained only if we assume that the insect has a 'scheme of things': that is, that its relations with its environment are not merely passive responses to external objects, but determined by its own purposes. Things around it have a *meaning* for it in relation to its purposes. But these purposes and this meaning are clearly not explicitly conscious – the insect does not have a language in which to make them explicit. They exist because there is a 'current of activity which flows towards the world', and which continues to flow through the tied, but not the amputated, limb. The insect is not passively responding to stimuli, but actively seeking to achieve its purposes in the world.

Regardless of what one thinks about this particular example, we can ask whether this makes sense as a general account of at least some of the behaviour of living organisms, including ourselves. In doing this, however, we should not misinterpret phrases like 'current of activity'. They could be taken as an expression of a discredited doctrine of 'vitalism', according to which living things are animated by a special, non-physical force, an *élan vital*, which makes their parts move in purposive ways. Merleau-Ponty makes it clear in his writings that he does not advocate any such doctrine. Just as a body-subject does not contain a mysterious, non-physical soul, responsible for thought, so it does not contain a mysterious, non-physical life-force responsible for its purposive movements. There is nothing more to the insect, or ourselves, than a living organism, composed of various chemical substances. Nevertheless, he would argue, there are aspects of the behaviour of a living organism, just as such, which require us to use concepts like 'meaning' and 'purpose' in their explanation. The aspects in question are just those which enable us to distinguish between a living organism and any non-living thing: they, as it were, follow from what we mean by 'alive'.

We do in fact distinguish between things which are alive and those which are not: things which are alive, for example, actively seek out food when, and because, they feel hungry, whereas nothing which is not alive can literally be said to seek out anything, or to feel anything. This means that the world, for the living but not the non-living being, can be said to pose a series of problems, which its activities are attempts to solve. Merleau-Ponty (2002: 90) compares the insect to something non-living like a drop of oil, which simply 'adapts itself to given external forces' – that is, whose movements are determined only by the character of the external situation in which it happens to be located. For instance, it may run down a piece of paper, and the direction of its movements will be determined simply by the way in which the paper is lying: it will, as we say, seek the line of least resistance – except that it *seeks* nothing, it just behaves as the situation makes it do. The insect, by contrast 'itself projects the norms of its environment and itself lays down the terms of its vital problem'. The insect has a world of its own – the world as perceived in relation to its needs and purposes; the drop of oil simply exists in *the* world, its behaviour shaped by things outside itself.

Neither the insect nor the drop of oil, Merleau-Ponty says (loc. cit.) exercises any choice. That is, neither of them acts on the basis of reflective thought: the drop of oil does not act at all, while the insect's actions are the result of what Merleau-Ponty calls 'an a priori of the species' – simply expressed, they are the result of blind instinct. Nevertheless, in the wider sense of choice identified above, the insect, unlike the oil-drop, can be said to choose. It does genuinely *act* rather than simply respond passively, and its actions are *its own*, part of its individual life, unlike the oil-drop's movements, governed by impersonal laws of cause and effect. In acting, it is pursuing its own purposes, which give it *reasons* for acting as it does and not in some other way. In this wider sense, some of our own behaviour can also be said to be chosen, that is, to be done for reasons, even though our reasons for choosing it are not made explicit. The applicability of concepts like choice, reason and purpose comes from the fact that it seems impossible fully to explain the behaviour except in these terms, that is, in terms of its meaning for us. The movements of a good footballer on the field of play are, most of the time, not explicitly thought out, but are nevertheless purposive: they cannot be explained except as attempts to achieve a certain purpose, such as to pass the ball to a member of one's own side who is in a good position to score a goal. If one could not explain them in that way, then one could not distinguish a well-placed pass from an accidental kick which just happened to direct the ball to a suitable player.

The difference between a human being and an insect is that most of our purposive actions, whether consciously thought out or not, are not the outcome of an 'a priori of the species'. The footballer's skill, though it may have roots in innate abilities, is the result of the development of those abilities by learning. Learning, in the sense required here, necessarily involves under-standing of relevant concepts, and it is the capacity to understand concepts – in a broad sense, to use language – which particularly distinguishes human beings from most other living organisms. It makes it possible, first, for us to have much more complex purposes, of the kind which need articulation in language. For example, we can have the purpose of canvassing for a political party, which is possible only if we have such complex concepts as 'political party', 'elections', 'voting' and 'canvassing'. Second, it makes it possible for individuals to have different purposes: the concepts I have formed and which identify my purposes can be different from those which you have. For these more sophisticated and individualized choices, perhaps we could speak of *deliberate* choice, which corresponds much more closely to the idealized model mentioned earlier.

What the footballer learns is how to play the ball in football – how to dribble, how to pass, how to kick goals, and so on: and this necessarily requires an understanding, first of all, of what football is, what the rules and point of the game are, and, then, of the component parts of the game – the concepts of dribbling, passing, goal-scoring, and so on. We can't sensibly offer a meaning-explanation of what he is doing as 'passing to his team-mate who is in a good position to score' unless it is true that he has a grasp of these concepts, but offering this meaning-explanation implies that he is *choosing* to kick the ball as he does, whether or not he is engaged in any conscious reflection on what he is doing.

Human development

If human subjectivity is essentially embodied, then it seems natural to say that it is capable of development in parallel with that of the body. Physically speaking, we start our lives as a cluster of cells, which becomes progressively more complex and organized until birth. In the prenatal, and in the immediate postnatal, phase, it makes little sense to explain any of our behaviour in terms of concepts. Concepts necessarily have to be learned, and learning takes time and experience. The behaviour of foetuses and neonates, therefore, while it may admit, in some of its aspects, of meaning-explanation, does so in much the same way as the behaviour of comparably complex non-human animals. The baby instinctively seeks out the breast; its eyes follow a light, and so on. Human life from then on develops through the progressive learning of more and more complex concepts, which is in part a matter of the assimilation of what were called, in an earlier chapter, human norms.

These more complex concepts, as was said above, are those which require language for their articulation. We learn concepts through learning to participate with other human beings in the collective activities in which those concepts figure, that is, in which the relevant terms are used. The more complex the concepts we acquire, the more complex the purposes we can have, and the more capable we become of making conscious and reflective choices – what were called above deliberate choices – and the acquisition of more complex concepts is naturally part of participation in more complex collective activities, that is, part of the process by which we develop from babies to children to adolescents to normal adults.

To say that this is a process of development is to say that the later stages build on the earlier. Earlier experiences are retained in the form of memories, whether explicit or implicit in the habits of behaviour which have been formed. This follows from the fact that human beings are in the world as subjects, not merely as objects. As subjects, we *experience* the world, rather than simply responding to it; and the character of our present experience is intelligible only in relation to what we have experienced in the past. It is only possible to speak of human beings as subjects at all to the extent that they have developed a first-person point of view – that is, have learned to identify themselves as 'I', and to distinguish between themselves and the world around them, including other selves. (This point of view can, and presumably must, pre-exist the actual use of the first-person pronoun). An experience is always *someone's* experience, so to speak of an experience it is necessary to be able to distinguish *my* experience both from other people's and from the objects which I experience. This distinction becomes more marked to the extent that I can relate my present experience to my own past. In this sense, my present experience is what it is only because I have had the past experiences I have had. We can be said to become who we are (a paradoxical form of words), as we develop more complex and differentiated selves in this way.

One of the implications of the view that human beings are body-subjects, however, is that their personhood – their existence as subjects – emerges from their pre-personal existence as bodies. 'Personal existence', Merleau-Ponty says, 'is intermittent' (Merleau-Ponty 2002: 97). Even in adulthood, we are conscious of ourselves as subjects only some of the time, and much of our activity is the outcome, not so much of instincts, as of habits of behaviour and response which were laid down in the past. These habits were originally established because they had some significance for us at the time, but have since become 'sedimented', to use Merleau-Ponty's word, in the body, part of the necessary impersonal background to our fully personal existence. Their sedimentation makes them more difficult to formulate explicitly, and so make them harder for ourselves or others to make rationally intelligible. He relates this to the Freudian concept of 'repression': '... we speak of repression in the limited sense', he says, (loc. cit.), 'when I retain through time one of the momentary worlds through which I have lived, and make it the formative element of my whole life'. Thus, I may in childhood for instance, have tried, in an infantile way, to solve the problem, as I saw it at the time, of my relation to one or other of my parents, or of reconciling my relation to one with that to the other. If I can now recall that problem and my solution, I can relate it to my present world – if only in seeing that that problem no longer exists for me, so that the solution is no longer relevant. It then becomes part of the normal way in which we construct ourselves as adults by taking up our past lives and incorporating them in some way into our present.

Suppose that something happened at the time which gave us a reason for *not* recalling that past situation. Suppose we encountered some obstacle which we did not have the strength to overcome. It might be, very plausibly, that the problem, as it presented itself to us at the time, just seemed too difficult for us to resolve – it was just too emotionally traumatic. Then we might remain 'imprisoned in the attempt and [use] up [our] strength indefinitely renewing it in spirit' (Merleau-Ponty 2002: 95). We should 'continue to be the person who ... once lived in this parental universe' (2002: 96). In other ways, we should continue with our development, incorporating into ourselves new experiences of various kinds: but this part of ourselves would remain, sedimented in our bodies, still the child, faced with this childish problem. Repression, Merleau-Ponty goes on:

> is the transition from first person existence to a sort of abstraction of that existence, which lives on a former experience ... [in this way, it is] an advent of the impersonal ... revealing our condition as incarnate beings by relating it to the temporal structure of being in the world.
>
> (Merleau-Ponty 2002: 96)

The idea of repression was connected by Freud, of course, with the origins of neurosis. For him neurosis arises, roughly speaking, from the conflict between what is repressed and the aims of the ego or I, the conscious adult self. In Merleau-Ponty's account of repression, then, we can see the possibility of one way in which the need for a meaning-explanation of mental disorder could perhaps be reconciled with the description of at least some mental disorders as mental illness. (To avoid misunderstanding, the point here is not to propose the correctness of the repression theory of the origins of mental illness, only to show how it might be logically possible to give a meaning-explanation of something that can be called an illness). Everything about the mental disorder would then be susceptible of a meaning-explanation – intelligible in terms of what the person was doing or attempting to do. The child was trying to solve an overwhelming emotional problem, and failing, with corresponding emotional trauma. This trauma gave the child a motive to 'forget' the attempt, but also a motive to keep on trying to resolve the problem. These continuing attempts would form part of the situation which confronted the adult in her attempts to form a coherent personality, capable of acting. The disorder in the adult would arise from the inevitable difficulty of this attempt at integration. All of this would be purposive, and in principle intelligible as such, but none of it would be the product of conscious deliberation, and so of choice in the narrow sense. It is as if the emerging personal self were invaded by its own impersonal background – almost from the outside, if not quite.

If this is a possible account of the origins of at least some of the typical mental disorders, it would allow us to call disorders of this type illnesses. They would still be different from bodily illnesses, which are straight forwardly caused by factors altogether outside self. Bodily illness is in a very straightforward sense something that *happens* to someone, and which is not directly subject to that person's own choice. Whereas this type of mental illness would be a distortion of one's own present choices by the continuing influence of one's past attempts to solve problems in one's personal life, which were chosen in the sense of being made for reasons, though not the outcome of conscious deliberation. This has a bearing, as I shall argue in a moment, on the kind of treatment which would be appropriate for such mental disorders, but it is not sufficient to make the term illness inapplicable to them.

What I have attempted to do in this account is to show how a pattern of *behaviour*, which must, as such, be explained in terms of the agent's reasons, could nevertheless qualify as an illness, something deserving help and compassion rather than either praise or condemnation. Whether this fits any particular disorders is a matter for empirical enquiry, not for a priori analysis: though it seems very plausible that one could explain some of the most typical mental disorders in this way. The account tries to do this by emphasizing the temporal or developmental nature of the human self, which is a consequence of our essential embodiment. What I am now, and so the reasons which have force for me now, are the product of what I have been in the past. That might suggest that my present self is the *causal* product of my past, but that suggestion would be misleading. What we might call normal development consists in a person's *learning from* past experience – for example, trying to solve problems in one's dealings with significant others, failing, and learning from that failure to adopt a different solution. Our essential embodiment means that these attempts at problem-solving and this learning need not be conscious, that is, explicitly formulated. But they can be, and, with increasing sophistication and linguistic capacity as we get older, they tend increasingly to be conscious, or to be based on conscious thought, and they can be more subtle. Difficulties arise when, for one reason or another – the strong emotions connected with particular problems, the lack of a sufficiently developed and sophisticated capacity to cope, or perhaps even the effects of brain damage – a past attempt at problem-solving becomes embedded in habits of response of which one is not conscious and so which is isolated from the normal path of development.

The similarities with Freud's account of the origins of neurosis have already been noted, and are anyway obvious, but similarities in the general structure of the account do not imply acceptance of all the details of Freudian theory. They do not commit us, for example, to Freud's emphasis on the central place of sexuality in human development and psychic life (though Merleau-Ponty himself is willing to go along with Freud in that respect: see Merleau-Ponty 2002: 178ff.). Given the conception of ourselves as body-subjects, there is a sense in which all our mental life must ultimately be rooted in our bodily needs. It may also be true that sexuality is more central to our sense of our own identity as persons than any other aspect of our embodiment. But it does not follow that all the problems we encounter in our development are in any meaningful sense sexual: for one thing, we have other bodily needs, and for another, the nature of a problem may be best understood, not in terms of its ultimate roots, but in terms of what has grown from those roots. Even if, for example, our relationship to our parents is rooted, as Freud suggests, in sexual desires, the problems which those relationships present us with might be best understood in terms of, say, our dependence on them for emotional and practical support rather than in specifically sexual terms.

For the same reason, we do not need to go along with Freud in seeing the origins of our adult psychological problems as lying exclusively in our early childhood. As far as this account goes, they need only to lie somewhere in our past, in attempted solutions which have become isolated from our general development as persons. The examples which Merleau-Ponty himself gives include problems in 'a love-affair, a career, a piece of work' (Merleau-Ponty 2002: 95) – all features of adult life, rather than of early childhood. Early childhood, it seems plausible to say, may well be the period in our lives when we are most likely, because of the underdevelopment of our mental resources, to become 'imprisoned in the attempt' to overcome such obstacles in our way, but again it does not follow that it is the only time when this can happen and so in which mental disorder of this kind can originate.

In one respect, however, the present account is essentially in accord with Freud, that is Freud's conception of the method of treating neurosis, namely psychotherapy. With some reservations, to be discussed later, our account of how this type of mental illness might be explained does imply that 'talking therapies' are central to its treatment. This follows from the conception of the nature of the disorder, as a problem in our being-in-the-world, rather than one resulting from the dysfunction or failure to function of some biological system. What the sufferer needs is to be helped to find some way of being-in-the-world which will not generate these problems. This is not, as Merleau-Ponty points out, a matter of making an intellectual discovery. Since the problem is not merely theoretical, it cannot be resolved by gaining a theoretical understanding of it: a problem in being-in-the-world can be resolved only by reorienting the way in which one is in the world. We have, as Merleau-Ponty puts it, to 'relive' the buried past as significant, 'and this the patient succeeds in doing only by seeing his past in the perspective of his co-existence with the doctor' (Merleau-Ponty 2002: 529). I interpret this to mean that the relationship with the psychiatrist constitutes a change in the way the patient is in the world, which enables the patient to reconceive themself in relationship to their own past. The origins of their problems are, as it were, exposed in their relationship to the therapist, and so it becomes possible for them to work out the problem in a conscious way, with all the mental resources of an adult, not as a merely intellectual exercise, but as an actual change in their life.

Mental illness, rationality, and the brain

There is, however, a danger of misunderstanding here, as Merleau-Ponty himself recognizes. If mental disorder is a distorted way of being-in-the-world, does that mean it is simply a 'problem in living', of the kind that Szasz speaks of? All human beings experience all sorts of problems in their attempts to cope with the world and other people. Relationships with others seldom run completely smoothly and often cause unhappiness – not to mention the more obviously existential problem of finding a path through life which will give us some sense of our activities as being meaningful. Is there really no difference between the kinds of problems which we classify as mental illness and the problems which we all have to deal with? It is increasingly the case in modern Western society that people seek the help of professional psychotherapists and counsellors in dealing with such existential problems. We live in what has been called a therapeutic culture, in which these problems are not regarded as moral or spiritual, to be dealt with judgmentally by such people as the clergy, but as sources of personal unhappiness, to be removed by therapists. It is not relevant to the themes of this book to consider whether this is a good or a bad development: but it is relevant to ask whether there is not a distinguishable category of problems which require something more like a medical approach, and, if so, what it is exactly which distinguishes them.

In some cases, as we have already seen, we can distinguish a category of disorders which, though undoubtedly mental in some sense, could not conceivably, at least in their core manifestations, be helped by psychotherapy, because they are the direct result of disturbances in the workings of the brain. The most obvious cases are those which consist in failures in normal mental *capacities*, such as the capacity to remember or the capacity to control one's own movements. Both of these are mental capacities in an ordinary sense of the term mental. Failure in either, moreover, leads to distortions in one's being-in-the-world. Inability to remember one's own past leads to loss of much of one's sense of one's own identity, and of the capacity to recognize others to whom one is related; failure to control one's own behaviour clearly leads to difficulties in coping with the world and other people. So by any criterion these are mental disorders, but also neurological conditions: as the latter, they clearly require medical intervention of standard kinds rather than talking therapies (though counselling can of course he helpful in alleviating the human consequences of the neurological incapacity). If it is the case, therefore, as it certainly seems to be, that the memory defects of Alzheimer's sufferers are a direct consequence of deterioration in brain tissue, then Alzheimer's is clearly a mental illness, not just a problem in living, but its treatment must be neurological, not psychotherapeutic. Similarly, if the tendency of some sufferers from Tourette's syndrome to utter obscenities in inappropriate places is a direct result of failures in normal control mechanisms, then Tourette's is, in this respect at least, an example of a mental illness which requires medical treatment rather than psychotherapy. Just because they can be adequately explained in neurological terms and treated by neurological means, such conditions might be better classified as neurological disorders than as forms of mental illness (this indicates some of the slipperiness of the notion of mental illness, which I shall return to at the end of the chapter).

Conditions on the autistic spectrum are usually described as mental disorders: but they do not seem on present understanding to admit of a meaning-explanation, and there is some evidence that they have a neurological, and perhaps a genetic origin. It is arguable, however, that it might be better to think of them as neither mental illness, nor as neurological disorders, but as part of a distinct category. Some autistic people do indeed campaign for greater social recognition of their distinctness: and say that what is need is not a cure for autism, but greater efforts to integrate autistic people and their distinctive ways of seeing the world into mainstream culture. The empirical evidence about their causation is at present unclear, and it would be inappropriate in a work such as this to seek to pre-empt future empirical investigation. But *if* it is the case that a certain way of behaving and reacting, such as autism, is largely genetically determined, and so cannot be treated medically, except perhaps by some form of gene therapy which would alter the person's genetic identity, then perhaps it should be thought of as a personality type rather than as a disorder. Having this personality type is liable to create problems for the person in coping with life in normal society, just as a mental disorder would, but it is not appropriate to speak of *treating* it. There is a role for a form of treatment which would consist in helping the autistic person, without ceasing to be who they are, to deal with some of the major problems which they will encounter in dealing with non-autistic people (the majority), but this would not be medical treatment in any ordinary sense: rather, it would be a form of social education. Even if autism turns out not to be a genetically determined condition, and to be treatable by more standard medical means, it is at least conceivable that there may be other ways of behaving currently classified as mental disorders which better fit the account given in this paragraph. Psychopathy might be a case in point, or personality disorders: it might be more illuminating and practically helpful to see them as unusual personality types, to be helped if they find difficulty in fitting in with life in normal society, but not to be medically treated, as if they were ill.

The connection of most other familiar types of mental disorder with brain deficiencies is, to say the least, not so obvious. Mood disorders such as depression seem to involve abnormalities of brain chemistry, and can be alleviated by pharmacological means. But it does not follow that they are directly *caused* by the problems in brain chemistry, in the way that loss of memory is caused by deterioration in brain structures. The existence of evidence that forms of psychotherapy such as cognitive behaviour therapy can also be helpful in cases of depression would in itself suggest that there is more to the explanation of depression than chemistry. This is reinforced by the fairly obvious connection in many cases between traumatic experiences, such as bereavement or the shocks of war, and the onset of depression. Depression, after all, is intentional: one is depressed *about something*. There is a difference, of course, between clinical depression and 'ordinary' depression. In normal life, we get depressed about something specific: about the failure of a relationship, or our lack of success in the world of work, or our financial problems. Finding a solution to those problems can then alleviate the depression. Those who are clinically depressed experience something much more all-pervasive and indeterminate, affecting their capacity for enjoyment, their sense of self-worth, their general vitality and so on. Nevertheless, an indeterminate object is still an object: depression is a state of mind which is not merely an inner experience, but is directed toward the outside world, whether it is the world in general or some specific aspect of it. In this sense, it requires some conception of how the world is – is it seen as depressing? It cannot be identified only with inner feelings, and so cannot be explained fully by the causes of those inner feelings.

The inner feeling of being depressed is common to ordinary depression, moderate clinical depression, and severe clinical depression. The differences between these forms are not simply matters of degree – though they are in part such. They are also differences of *kind*. Ordinary depression is understandable: that is, we can readily imagine why someone should feel depressed in their situation, even if we have never been in that situation ourselves, and even if we might make a more resilient response to it if we were. Because of this, we can give a complete explanation of the depressed mood as a response to this situation: the mood is not something which (causally) explains the depression, but a part of the depresssion which is to be explained. In clinical cases, on the other hand, there is either no obvious reason in the external situation to explain the mood, or else the external reason scarcely seems to justify the depth of the mood or its impact on the rest of the person's life. The 'reasons' which may be offered therefore may come to seem more like *rationalizations*. The inner mood comes to occupy central place: it is something which seems to come and go in a way which is inexplicable in terms of reasons. The explanatory weight therefore comes to fall more on the causes of the mood which is being rationalized in this way – but this seems to contradict what was said in the preceding paragraph, at least as far as clinical depression is concerned. Is there any way in which this impasse can be avoided?

We can perhaps find some help in Merleau-Ponty's discussion of the Freudian conception of the all-pervasiveness of sexuality in human life – a good example of the usefulness of the idea of human beings as body-subjects. Using it in this way does not imply that we have to accept the full-blown Freudian theory of sexuality. Its point is only to illustrate the way in which the notion of human beings as body-subjects enables us to conceive of the relation between causal and meaning explanation, giving due weight to each and to their interaction. We can note first that the most obvious way to define sexuality is in terms of genital activity and the thoughts and feelings associated with it. If the term sexual is to have any meaning, it might be thought, then (as with any other term) it must be possible to distinguish what is sexual from what is not, and how else could we do that? So to speak of sexuality as being all-pervasive in the way that Freud does seems to deprive the term of any specific meaning: a sexuality which pervades every aspect of human existence seems to be little more than a synonym for existence itself, so that 'all human existence is sexual' seems to mean no more than the tautology that 'all human existence is human existence'. Sexuality thus seems to be reduced to something vague and spiritual: its distinctive carnality seems to be lost.

Nevertheless, Merleau-Ponty argues, there does seem to be some meaning to talk of sexuality as such pervading every aspect of human life. What that meaning is, he attempts to bring out by use of the concept of the body-subject. To say that human beings are body-subjects, as was said earlier, is to say both that bodily movements and processes and needs have to be understood in terms of subjective meanings, and that subjective meanings have to be understood against the background of bodily movements, processes and needs. We can neither reduce human existence to the workings of a bodily machine nor reduce the workings of the body to expressions of the human spirit. There is, in Merleau-Ponty's words, a 'dialectical' relationship between body and subject – a kind of conversation between them, in which they reciprocally influence each other.

Thus, in relation to sexuality, such phenomena as modesty, desire and love have a 'metaphysical significance, which means that they are incomprehensible if man is treated as a machine governed by natural laws' (Merleau-Ponty 2002: 193). We cannot explain, he is arguing, why a human being should feel uncomfortable about showing her body to a stranger in terms of the laws of physics and chemistry: the explanation, if it is to work, must be in terms of how she experiences her own body, as something which can be seen by others as an object, but which she herself wants to be seen as an expression of her subjectivity. At the same time, we should not have such feelings at all if we did not have bodies of the kinds which we do, including sexual organs and urges which force upon us the kinds of relationships with others in which feelings of modesty, desire and sexual love play an essential part. Because our personal existence emerges against the background of our existence as living bodies, it is inevitably pervaded by an atmosphere generated by the nature of that bodily existence. In simpler terms, modesty, desire and love can be understood in terms of their subjective significance, but also have preconditions which depend on bodily functioning, that is, biology.

Can we apply this to the case of depression? Depression, we might say first of all, is a permanently possible way in which human beings can respond to the world – one which is inherent in the way in which human brain chemistry works. This response is normally provoked straightforwardly by surrounding life-events – say, the loss of someone very near and dear. But such life-events make us depressed – that is, our reaction to them is expressed in this sort of mood, because our bodies are structured in certain ways. If we were differently made, then we might not experience bereavement at all, as we know it, or, if we did, our response to bereavement might take a different form. In this sense, we can give both a meaning-explanation in terms of a response to life-events and a causal explanation of the underlying predisposition to such a response which is implicit in human biology.

In some cases, however, what is distinctive is that most of us do not feel able to give a meaning-explanation in terms of normally expected reasons for being depressed, and so treat the mood as a purely natural phenomenon, requiring only a causal explanation. But it clearly does not follow from the fact that we do not feel able to give a meaning-explanation that no meaning-explanation can in principle be given. Indeed, the suggestion above was that, if we are to call the mood one of depression, we must be able, in principle, to find a meaning-explanation for it. Perhaps we are just too unimaginative, too hidebound by conventional ideas of what is intelligible, or even too lazy. In many cases of clinical depression, a meaning-explanation can be found, and this is what is worked on in psychotherapy. Because this is not a normal situation, we need to find a particular kind of explanation, however: there is thus a further question as to why the person is particularly prone to find things in her situation depressing, and so would be likely both to respond to elements which most people would not find such and to respond to them in a more all-embracing way than normal. This explanation would presumably lie in something distinctive about her biochemistry, which intensified the common human disposition to respond depressively to certain kinds of situation. In such a case, the biological explanation of the predisposition would suggest ways in which pharmacological treatment would alleviate the mood and so make it more possible for psychotherapy to be effective. In cases of very severe depression, it might of course be that pharmacological alleviation of this kind was all that could in practice be done to help the patient.

Some aspects of some other recognized mental disorders could be analysed in similar ways. One example might be the delusions which are a characteristic feature of schizophrenia, and indeed of other forms of mental illness. Not all delusions are false beliefs, as Fulford has reminded us, and not all are factual beliefs at all: we can also make delusional value judgements (Fulford 1989: 203 ff.). To use Fulford's own examples: a man can be deluded in thinking his wife is unfaithful to him, even though his wife is indeed having an affair with someone else; and we can be deluded in feeling ourselves to be worthless, or guilty of grave sin, or conversely in feeling ourselves to be god-like in our powers. It is well to be reminded of this if we are to avoid over-simplified explanations of delusion.

What makes these beliefs and value judgements delusions and contrasts them with normal beliefs, true or false, or normal value judgements, commonplace or otherwise, is surely the role which they play in the deluded person's way of being-in-the-world. This is not a matter of being irrational in one sense of that term: many of the beliefs that most of us hold, and of the value judgements that most of us make, are irrational in the sense that they have no rationally adequate grounds. The person who holds the beliefs or makes the value judgements does not do so as the result of careful consideration of the evidence or arguments for or against, but because they seem emotionally satisfying or pragmatically convenient. Human beings have a natural tendency to jump to conclusions, usually motivated by emotion rather than evidence. The delusions of the mentally ill are no different in that respect: but the emotions which they satisfy or the pragmatic purposes for which they are useful are disordered, in the sense of being unintelligible, or intelligible only with great difficulty, by most members of society. The man who believes his wife to be unfaithful is deluded, not because that belief is necessarily false, but because suspicion of his wife's loyalty to him is a part of a sense of his own vulnerability. This unusual sense of vulnerability may well be explicable causally, in biochemical terms (though it may equally well be the result of early experiences which he has had): but even if biochemistry does explain the vulnerability, it does not suffice to explain why it is expressed in this particular belief rather than others. Belief is intentional: what makes it this belief is that it is *about* his wife and her relationship to him. So what needs to be explained about the belief is why it is about this rather than about anything else, and that demands a meaning-explanation: what purpose does it serve in the man's scheme of things? Treatment of delusions, likewise, involves both trying to deal (perhaps by medication, or perhaps by psychotherapy) with the sources of the man's sense of vulnerability, and (certainly by psychotherapy) dealing with the reasons why he feels particularly vulnerable in his relations with his wife.

As a final example, we might consider a phobia, such as agoraphobia. Fear of certain kinds of situations is, again, a feature of human beings as embodied creatures. There are no doubt good evolutionary reasons why a tendency to be afraid of open spaces, in particular, should be built into human biology. People with agoraphobia have this fear to an unusual, and incapacitating, extent: but, like normal fear, it is identified as what it is by its intentional object, namely, open spaces. What makes this a disorder is that the fear cannot be justified in terms which others would find readily intelligible, but it does not follow that it cannot be given a meaning-explanation. Just because fear, even irrational fear, is intentional, it must be possible to find reasons why it should be directed to this object rather than any other: why does the person fear open spaces, and not, say, snakes or darkness? No biochemical investigation could answer this question, since the biochemistry of fear is the same whatever the intentional object may be. What biochemistry can explain is why this person might be more liable than most to feel fear in their situation, and so might be predisposed to having irrational fears. If so, then the treatment of phobias must be primarily directed to dealing with the unusual reasons for fear, that is, it must be psychotherapeutic, but there is still a role for pharmacological treatments in controlling the underlying predisposition.

Some conclusions about mental illness

We have now reached the completion of the general philosophical analysis of the idea of mental illness and the relevance of the medical model. In the remaining two chapters, I shall consider some legal and ethical issues in the light of this analysis. Before I do so, it may be helpful to try to summarize, fairly briefly, what has been said so far. The ideas of mental disorder and mental illness have turned out to be slippery – that is, their meaning is hard to pin down, so that it is hard to decide just what counts as a mental disorder, just where the boundaries lie between one mental disorder and another, and just where the limits of applicability of the whole concept should be drawn.

There are similar problems with the idea of the medical model. I have tried to show how a traditional view of medicine (at least since Descartes) saw it as an application of scientific knowledge (drawn ultimately from physics and chemistry) to the manipulation of a certain kind of object, namely, the human body, conceived of as a certain kind of machinery. The values which determined to what ends that manipulation should take place were supplied by the human beings to whom that machinery belonged. They (or most of them) wanted to stay alive as long as possible, to be able to engage in certain kinds of activities, to be free of excessive pain, and so on. The job of the medical profession was then to use their knowledge of the body to correct its workings when it got into a state in which people might be liable to premature death, inefficiency in performing desirable activities, and excessive pain.

The medical model in this sense does not seem to fit very well with human mental life. Our thoughts, feelings, moods, desires and so on are not parts of some external machinery, loosely attached to us and capable of affecting our lives in the undesirable ways mentioned. They are *us*, and vice versa. To call them disordered is not to equate them with biological malfunctions which limit our life and activity, but to say that in respect of them our life and activity are themselves going wrong in some way. We might put it in this way: in bodily disorders, it is our bodies which are not working properly; in mental disorders, we ourselves are not living properly. Bodily disorder transgresses biological norms; mental disorder deviates from what I have called human norms. We can thus agree at least to some extent with Christopher Boorse, in that we can share his feeling that mental disorder is not illness in exactly the same sense as bodily illness. It is a sickness in our *experience* of the world.

Here, however, there are further complications. The distinction between mental and bodily disorder still depends too much on Cartesian dualism. Bodily illness too affects our way of being-in-the-world: if we are ill, especially if we are very ill, this necessarily has an impact not only biologically but also humanly – we react differently to other people and the world in general. On the other hand, mental disorders necessarily have biological (especially neurological) correlates, and can yield, to some extent at least, to physical treatments – medication, even surgery. And they have a bearing on our biological efficiency: people die prematurely from suicide as well as from cancer.

I have suggested that, to cope with these problems, we need to abandon Cartesian dualism and to substitute for it Merleau-Ponty's conception of human beings as body-subjects. The mind is then not thought of, as in dualism and even in classical materialism, as a 'thing' which constitutes one part of a human being. Rather, human beings are thought of as wholes, who exist in the world and whose bodies (including their brains) are experienced as their means of existing in the world. What happens to my body happens to me, and the purposes which I have are expressed in the movements of my body. The most that one can say, on this view, is that bodily and mental disorder are distinguished in so far as we can separate (as in practice we usually can) the ways in which my being-in-the-world is affected, on the one hand, by the shortening of my lifespan, the enfeeblement of my activity and the effects of pain, from those in which it is affected by the distortion of my personal relations to others and to things. And only some mental disorders in this sense can qualify, I have argued, as full-blown mental illnesses, for which something like medical treatment is appropriate: namely, those which involve suffering for the person concerned because, in one way or another, they are not deliberately chosen by that person.

Once we accept that mind is not the name of a thing, but of aspects of human activities, then we can also accept that these activities are very varied in character. Thinking is a different way of relating to the world from feeling, and both from wishing, desiring and so on. Again, when we talk about someone's mind, we sometimes refer to certain of their capacities, and sometimes to the experiences which they have. Thoughts can be disordered in different ways from feelings; capacities in different ways from experiences. Thus, as I have tried to show in this chapter, we should not think of mental disorders, or even all mental illnesses as of a piece: as if the concept of mental disorder applied to a homogeneous class of human conditions. The standard classifications such as DSM-IV and ICD-10, for good pragmatic reasons, list a whole range of very different conditions, and divide them up into distinct diagnostic categories. In reality the differences become clear: some mental disorders, or perhaps rather some elements in what are called mental disorders, are failures of capacities, and as such have similarities to bodily diseases, both in their explanation and in their treatment. Some are more comparable to personality types. Some are explainable mainly in terms of a person's reasons for acting or responding in that way, which neither, as I argued earlier, excludes thinking of them as illness nor precludes the limited relevance of physical treatment. To ask the question, 'Does the medical model apply to mental disorder?' is too simple: it glosses over both the complexity of the notion of mental disorder and the vagueness of the concept of the medical model. All this is relevant, as I shall now try to show, to a number of key ethical and legal issues connected with mental illness.

Chapter 7

Mental disorder and legal responsibility

Mad or bad?

It is true, almost by definition, that I can be held responsible only for what I have myself intentionally done (and conversely that I must be held responsible for all my own intentional actions). I clearly am not responsible for what someone else has done: if I had a twin brother, for instance, it would obviously be wrong to punish me for his crimes. And I am not responsible for things which I do not in any real sense 'do' – for things which just happen to me in ways which I cannot control, or for things which are the genuinely unforeseeable consequences of what I do. If my nose suddenly starts to bleed uncontrollably, then it would hardly be fair to blame me for the mess which that makes on your carpet; or if, in trying to make my way through an unfamiliar house in the dark, I accidentally brush against a precious vase, causing it to fall to the ground and break in pieces, it would be harsh to condemn me for my vandalism. If a court of law is trying to determine guilt or innocence, then the first question to ask is, 'Is the accused the person who actually did the crime?'; and the second, assuming the answer to the first is 'Yes', is, 'Did the accused intend to do it, or was he involved only by accident or as a result of factors beyond his control?' If the second alternative of the latter question is chosen, we are asserting that he did it, but that his action was excusable.

The business both of blaming and of excusing from blame is an inevitable part of normal human relationships, as the late Peter Strawson argued in his classic British Academy lecture, 'Freedom and Resentment' (Strawson 2003). Typical human relationships, constituting a human community, are based on mutual recognition: my attitudes to you depend on my perception of your attitudes to me. Strawson calls these 'reactive attitudes', those in which we respond to the perceived intentions and feelings of others towards ourselves. We feel resentment, for instance, when someone else does us an injury, if we perceive the injury as what he intended, but we modify our response if we come to see the action as not, on this occasion, meant to be injurious: 'The agent was just ignorant of the injury he was causing, or had lost his balance through being pushed or had reluctantly to cause the injury for reasons which acceptably override his reluctance' (Strawson 2003: 78). In those circumstances, we excuse the injury, but this forgiveness is itself a kind of reactive attitude – a reaction to the agent's intentions in action. We are still treating the person as a human being whose actions can be understood – a part of the human community.

Strawson's criteria of excusability can be traced back as far as Aristotle. In his *Nicomachean Ethics* 1109b30ff (Aristotle 2004: 50f.), Aristotle gives an account of what makes an action involuntary – still an action, but not one for which the agent can be blamed. Moral theorists and legislators, Aristotle sees, need to decide the limits of the voluntary – actions that 'receive praise and blame' – and the involuntary – actions that 'receive pardon and sometimes pity too'. The essence of his definition of the involuntary is: 'Actions are regarded as involuntary when they are performed under compulsion or through ignorance' (Aristotle 2004: 50). An action is performed under compulsion, according to Aristotle, 'when it has an external origin of such a kind that the agent or patient contributes nothing to it' (*ibid.*): his examples are of a voyager in a boat being conveyed by the wind, or of someone being forced to do something by others who had him in their power. There may be borderline cases, as Aristotle accepts. For instance, we may debate whether someone is acting voluntarily if they do something for fear of something worse: his example is of someone who obeys a tyrant who threatens to kill his children if he did not do as instructed. This kind of action is not, strictly speaking, done under compulsion: the man in the example does have a choice, but it would be unreasonable and inhuman to expect him to act otherwise. So, Aristotle concludes, such actions 'seem more like voluntary than involuntary ones … because at the time they are performed they are matters of choice' (*ibid.*). We might nevertheless feel that it would be inhuman to blame someone for doing what they did in such circumstances, even though in a sense they are fully responsible for their actions.

Turning to the other criterion, that of ignorance, Aristotle says that he has in mind 'not ignorance in the choice (this is a cause of wickedness), nor ignorance of the universal (for this people are blamed), but *particular* ignorance [italics in the original], i.e. of the circumstances and objects of the action' (Aristotle 2004: 53). What this seems to mean can be gathered from the context. 'Ignorance in the choice' appears to mean 'ignorance of what is right and wrong', and this is not supposed to excuse: indeed, it is 'a cause of wickedness'. Someone who behaves badly not knowing that they are behaving badly seems to be at least as open to blame as anyone else, at least if we can say that they ought to have known this. What makes an action involuntary, and so pardonable, for Aristotle is a different kind of ignorance – ignorance of what one is doing. Someone may know what they are doing under one description, but not under another: for instance, may know that they are revealing information, but not know that they are disclosing a secret. Others of Aristotle's examples (slightly adapted) are: mistaking the identity of someone he is attacking, as when someone thinks he is attacking an enemy but is really attacking someone completely innocent; thinking he was throwing a spear protected by a button (in a practice throw, for example), when actually the spear is unprotected, and so kills or injures someone; or administering a drug which he thought was life-saving, when in fact it was lethal. The mark of excusability about this ignorance, for Aristotle, is that the person in question feels distress and remorse when he discovers his mistake. This shows that they did not intend to do what they have in fact done, but something quite different. (Again one might say that much depends on whether we would *expect* them to have known: a pharmacist, for example, might be regarded as guilty of negligence if they didn't know that a drug was lethal).

There is a deep-rooted sense that mental derangement constitutes an excuse. If someone does something outrageously wrong, especially, we may suspect that they were mad rather than bad – not really to blame for what they did, because they 'couldn't help it'. This intuition is reflected in legal systems, most of which recognize what is often called an insanity defence. In those legal systems based on the common law tradition, the most often-cited statement of the criteria used in such a defence are the 'M'Naghten Rules'. These rules were first formulated in 1843 by the judges in the case of one Daniel M'Naghten (whose name has different spellings in different accounts), who was tried for shooting dead the private secretary of the then British Prime Minister, Robert Peel. M'Naghten suffered from the delusion that he was being persecuted by members of Peel's party, the Tories, and mistakenly took the private secretary to be Peel, perceived by him as his chief persecutor. This was the basis for a successful defence on the grounds of diminished responsibility because of insanity: the rules are an attempt to express the reasons for the success of this defence in this case. The judges said:

> To establish a defence on the grounds of insanity, it must be conclusively proved that, at the time of the committing of the act, the party accused was labouring under such a defect of reason, from the disease of the mind, as not to know the nature and quality of the act he was doing; or if he did know it, that he did not know what he was doing was wrong.

(quoted from Moore 1984: 218ff., with spellings Anglicized)

As has often been pointed out, the judges' tests bear a striking similarity in some ways to Aristotle's criteria of involuntariness, though they do not make any mention of the act's being done 'under compulsion', and they differ from Aristotle in thinking of ignorance of the wrongness of one's actions as an excuse. (Other legal formulations lay more emphasis on the idea of compulsion, and I shall return to this criterion shortly). The closest resemblance to Aristotle is on the criterion of ignorance of 'the nature and quality of the act he was doing'. Now, in one sense, because of the very nature of action, it is impossible to perform an action without knowing what one is doing. An action is identified by the description under which it falls, and the agent is only performing a particular action if they can identify it in that way. For instance, the same movements of the hand can fall under the description 'signing a cheque' and 'doodling on a piece of paper'. Which of these actions someone is performing depends on how he or she would describe what they are doing. If they have no idea what a cheque is, for example, then they simply cannot be said to be signing a cheque, however much their hand-movements may resemble those of someone who is genuinely performing that action. It follows that no one can sign a cheque without knowing that that is what he is doing.

In that sense, Daniel M'Naghten must have known what he was doing. He must have known he was shooting someone – otherwise what he was doing would not have been describable in that way. Quite apart from that logical point, he clearly had an intention to kill Peel, for reasons which he could have explained to others if he had been asked. So in any ordinary sense, he knew what he was doing as well as any 'sane' assassin, like one of the conspirators who attempted to assassinate Adolf Hitler to try to bring peace with the Allies and end the persecution of the Jews and others. Why therefore should M'Naghten be any less responsible for his actions than they were? (His mistaken identification of the private secretary was of course, irrelevant: it is no less culpable to kill the secretary than to kill his employer).

We might turn to Aristotle's examples and suggest that perhaps he didn't know what he was doing in the sense that there was a true description of what he was doing which he did not know, and which was relevant to determining guilt or innocence. Perhaps we might say that he knew he was shooting someone, but not that he knew he was shooting someone innocent of any harm towards him. He saw himself as acting in self-defence, we might say, rather than committing a murder: Peel, in his view, was intent on killing him and the shooting of the man he thought was Peel was a kind of pre-emptive strike. So he didn't know what he was doing in the sense that he didn't know that this was an act of murder, not of self-defence. For Aristotle, however, as was said earlier, the use of this excuse depends on whether the perpetrator feels distress or remorse on learning of the mistake. There is no evidence that

M'Naghten had any such feelings, or even acknowledged that he was mistaken in his view of Peel. The fact is that this was not a straightforward mistake, anyway, but a *delusion*, an unshakeable belief resulting from his 'disease of the mind'. But why should that be an excuse? It might be that, because of his delusion, he could not be *expected* to know the correct description of what he was doing: that would be the excuse, rather than the ignorance itself.

Part of the reason why insanity has been thought to be a defence seems to lie in traditional popular ideas of madness, for which insanity is the more respectable-sounding legal synonym. 'Mad' people are traditionally seen as those who have completely lost their reason (cf. the judge's phrase 'defect of reason, from the disease of the mind'). In that sense, they are not part of the general human community, in which we can see what reasons someone has for what they are doing, even when they are doing something wrong. To have reasons for what one is doing is to be in control of one's actions: so to lose one's reason is to lose one's powers of control over one's own behaviour – to act wildly and unpredictably, in the way non-human animals may do, and to be, like animals, not amenable to rational persuasion to do otherwise. Temporary insanity is also possible, as when someone in the grip of powerful emotions, such as anger or jealousy, loses control: they are, as we say, 'beside themselves' with rage or whatever. Madness is supposed to be the chronic version of this state: the great English philosopher of the seventeenth century, John Locke, describes the mad man as 'not himself' or 'beside himself' (Locke 1975: II.xxvii.20).

This suggests that madness, in this sense, offers a different kind of excuse from those listed by Aristotle. The mad person is seen as not really *acting* in the full sense at all, but as being the mere plaything of external forces. Sometimes these external forces were conceived as demons, which needed to be driven out by prayer or similar intervention if the mad person were to be restored to ordinary humanity. Sometimes mad people were seen as having become like wild animals, and so no longer subject to Reason, like human beings, but as governed by animal passions. In the latter case, their behaviour was now subject to external forces, but they had got themselves into this dehumanized condition by their own choice, to indulge in animal excess rather than to live by Reason. Hence, they needed punitive treatment to redeem them from their bestiality. (See Porter [2002] for a fascinating historical account of ideas of madness). Many of these ideas still survive, perhaps in attenuated form, in the present day, in tabloid headlines about the 'sick perverts' who commit horrendous crimes and are often explicitly called 'animals' or 'beasts'. But it would be irrational either to condemn or to excuse, say, a hungry lion who kills a child: both condemnation and forgiveness belong to the realm of human dealings with other human beings – the realm of Strawson's 'reactive attitudes'. People are excused, by Aristotle's criteria, if they did not really *mean* to do the wrong thing which they did: but animals cannot be said to mean to do things in this sense – they just *do* them, impelled, as we say, by their natural instincts. Those possessed by demons, even more obviously, neither mean nor do not mean to do what they do: it is the demons that act through them.

In his lecture, Strawson discusses a different kind of attitude which we may take. Sometimes, he says, we adopt what he calls 'objective attitudes'. These attitudes apply to a subgroup of cases which 'presents the agent as psychologically abnormal – or as morally undeveloped. The agent was himself; but he is warped or deranged, neurotic or just a child' (Strawson 2003: 79). Whereas reactive attitudes 'belong to involvement or participation with others in interpersonal human relationships', objective attitudes to someone are appropriate when 'you cannot reason with him' (ibid.). Strawson's picture of our normal involvement with others, as stated above, is of relations based on responses to each other's perceived intentions, and it is in that context that both resentment and forgiveness have some meaning. But when we cannot reason with someone else, then our relations with them must have some other basis: the implication is that they become something less than fully human, like animals, with whom also we cannot reason.

> To adopt the objective attitude to another human being is to see him, perhaps, as an object of social policy; as a subject for what, in a wide range of sense, might be called treatment; as something... to be managed or handled or cured or trained.
>
> (Strawson 2003: ibid.)

If Strawson is right, then the insanity defence makes sense. If being insane is (as traditional concepts of madness suggest) being less than fully human, being as impossible to reason with as the beasts of the field, then to commit an offence while suffering from a defect of reason is neither to be guilty nor to be excusable. A dog who attacks a baby is not brought to trial for the offence and acquitted on the grounds of dimished responsibility: it is either put down, or perhaps sent for retraining so that it will not offend in the same way in future. In somewhat the same way, the implication of Strawson's argument seems to be, a psychologically abnormal person who commits what would normally be a crime ought to be neither condemned nor excused, but given treatment (in less civilized times, it might even have been suggested that mad offenders ought to be put down).

It is interesting, however, that Strawson does not use the term mad, but the more scientific sounding term 'psychologically abnormal' (or even neurotic). Madness is not, and cannot be, part of the vocabulary of a psychiatry which has any pretensions to being scientific. For one thing, it is much too vague, indeed indefinable – its use is coloured far too much by personal emotions and valuations. For another, to call someone's behaviour or thinking mad is to imply that it is inexplicable in any empirically testable way – it is due to demonic possession or to an even more mysterious slide into animality: whereas to approach human behaviour scientifically it is necessarily to see it as explicable. People who, in scientific terms, are psychologically abnormal are still fully human, but have deviated from normal human patterns of thought and behaviour in ways which anyone else could have done in the same circumstances. The modern conception of an insanity defence, as exemplified in the M'Naghten tests, is a recognition of this, attempting to adapt the Aristotelian notion of involuntariness to modern notions of mental illness, as opposed to madness.

The trouble with this is that it is not clear, as already hinted, that mentally ill thought and action can be fitted into Aristotelian notions of involuntariness. It is not so much, for example, that a mentally ill offender 'does not know what he is doing', as that his way of conceiving what he is doing is different from what might seem natural to a more normal person. M'Naghten (knowingly) shoots the man he thought was the Prime Minister, because he sees that as an act of pre-emptive self-defence. So he knows the 'nature and quality' of his action under one description, but not under another. The question of responsibility thus seems, as suggested earlier, to turn on whether he could, given his delusion, have been expected to realize the incorrectness of this second description. This seems to be essentially an empirical question: it is certainly not a logically necessary truth, as far as one can see, that someone who has a deluded perception of himself and his situation is totally beyond the reach of rational persuasion, and so cannot be expected to think otherwise. The judges also stressed the importance of deciding whether the offender lacked an understanding of right and wrong: but cold-blooded murder was probably as repugnant for M'Naghten as the rest of us. He was not like a child, or a morally undeveloped adult, who could not reasonably be expected to know about the moral distinction between murder and killing in self-defence. His problem was not in his knowledge of right and wrong, but in his view of what he had done as self-defence. We could certainly reason with him (as we could not with an animal) about the morality of killing, but what we could almost certainly not convince him of by argument was that what he was doing was not morally justifiable.

The notion of psychosis is probably as close as scientific psychiatry comes to traditional ideas of madness: but of course the modern conception of mental illness has a much wider scope, and that creates further difficulties for attempts to formulate the insanity defence. People who suffer from sexual preference disorders, for example, may well have little in common with people who would traditionally have been described as mad. They may well act calmly, coldly, efficiently in pursuit of their goals: but those goals themselves may appear to most normal people to be, not simply, criminal but monstrous – for instance, the sexual abuse of small children. It is even more clearly the case with them than it was with M'Naghten that they know what they are doing. They may deceive themselves about the wrongness of what they are doing, but then, as we saw earlier, for Aristotle that was not a sign of involuntariness but, on the contrary, of greater wickedness. They may perhaps plead that they are acting under compulsion, but then they are using that expression in a different sense from Aristotle's, who confined it, as we saw, to compulsion by *external* forces: no one and nothing outside themselves appears to be *making* them act as they do. So in Aristotelian terms, they do not seem to be excusable.

Is determinism the answer?

Some might want to argue that we should follow up the implications of something said earlier – that any psychiatry with pretensions to being scientific holds human behaviour, including disordered behaviour, to be explicable in empirically testable ways. If we do that, they might say, we might see that it is a necessary truth that mentally ill people cannot be expected to behave, or indeed to think, otherwise than they do. The argument would go something like this: a scientific approach to the world, or to any part of it, presupposes a belief that everything that happens can be explained – a belief which is often identified with acceptance of universal determinism. Determinism, briefly expressed, is the doctrine that every event (i.e. everything which happens) has a cause. If a leaf falls from a tree in autumn, that is not to be seen as an inexplicable mystery, but as something whose causes (a combination in this case) can be traced: the wind blew, the attachment of the leaf to the tree was weakened, so that the wind caused the leaf to break off the branch, and the Earth's gravity caused it then to float down to the ground below. (Gravity might be described as a standing condition in this situation, rather than an immediate cause.) All these causes regularly act in this way in these circumstances, as can be established by empirical evidence, and that is all we need to know in order to understand what made the leaf fall in that way just then. Furthermore, the immediate causes themselves have causes, something which explains them in the same way: we can find a cause for the wind blowing in that place at that time, for the weakening of the leaf's attachment to the branch, and so on.

And these causes of causes themselves have causes, and so on back to the beginning of time. Thus, the thesis of universal determinism is that everything that happens in nature is part of a single, though immensely complex, causal nexus.

'Everything that happens in nature' includes, of course, human actions: so, if universal determinism is accepted, human actions must also have causes. The immediate cause of a human action may, consistently with determinism, be a choice, if that means only that something happened in the person's mind, or brain, which led to them doing what they did. For example, I might have written these words because I had the thought of writing these words, but then the thought itself, if determinism is true, must have a cause: why did I have that thought then? And the cause of my having that thought then must have a cause, and so on. Sooner or later, the chain of causes must cease to contain anything recognizable as a thought of my own, so that ultimately, the determinist would argue, what caused me to write these words was not the thought but something outside me which caused me to think in that way.

Philosophers dispute whether determinism is or is not compatible with free will and therefore with responsibility for one's actions: those who believe it is are, for obvious reasons, called 'compatibilists', and those who disagree are called, for equally obvious reasons, 'incompatibilists'. Which answer one gives largely depends on what one means by 'free will'. On one interpretation (compatibilist), to say that someone acts from free will, and so is responsible for what they have done, is to say that the immediate determining cause of the action is the person's own choice: this is perfectly compatible with determinism. On the opposing view, to say that a person has acted from free will would be to say that their action had *no* cause, which would clearly be incompatible with determinism as it is usually defined. Incompatibilists, however, could argue in their own favour that, whatever the immediate cause of the action may be, if that itself is determined by prior causes (which is, as just argued, required by determinism), then the *ultimate* cause of the action is not the person's choice, but something outside the person's own control. So compatibilist free will is not really free will at all: if determinism is true, free will does not exist, and, if responsibility for one's actions depends on free will, then responsibility does not exist either. If determinism is true, then *every* human action is done under compulsion in the strict Aristotelian sense, because every action is ultimately caused by something external to the agent.

Does this resolve the problem about the responsibility of those with mental illness? A scientific psychiatry aims to explain the peculiar thoughts, emotions and desires that mentally ill people have, and the peculiar behaviour which those thoughts, emotions and desires lead them to go in for. If we accept determinism, that means that everyone of these mental phenomena must have a cause, just like everything else in the universe, and so the search for an explanation must it seems amount to a search for such causes. Daniel M'Naghten's action in shooting Peel's secretary, for instance, was caused by his perception of this man as a potential threat to his own life. In that sense, he knew what he was doing, as Aristotle's criteria require. Furthermore, it looks at first sight at least that it was this *internal* thought of his which caused him to pull the trigger, not something obviously external to him: so his action was not, in Aristotle's terms, done under compulsion. But if we try to look into the example more scientifically, we shall ask what caused him to have this peculiar perception. It is so peculiar that it was clearly not caused in the same way as a sane person's perception that this was the Prime Minister's secretary, and an innocent man. The sane person's perception was caused, presumably, in part by the light rays entering his eyes and impinging on the retina, and then by this information's being processed by the person's brain in the usual way, connected with memories of previous experiences of Peel, etc. M'Naghten's deluded perception must have had some different cause: maybe peculiarities in his brain processes, or perhaps traumatic previous experiences. These other causes were what ultimately made him pull the trigger, not his immediate thought. So in a way, he was acting under compulsion, since what he was doing was really caused, not by what he *thought* he was doing, but by these ultimately external factors which caused him to have that thought. Even his perception of his action as self-defence must have been a result of the same causes, and so was equally compelled. So he couldn't be expected to think or act otherwise than he did, and wasn't really responsible for his action.

We can generalize this example. If we are to take a scientific approach to mental illness, the argument is, then we must assume that we can give a causal explanation of mentally ill thoughts and behaviour, but that means that the ultimate cause of what mentally ill people do is not a matter of their own choice, but of what causes them to choose as they do. This is why we do not hold mentally ill people to be responsible for their actions, and that is the basis for the insanity defence. It is as unfair to blame a mentally ill person for committing something which would normally be regarded as a crime as it would be to blame a slate for sliding off a roof and causing head injuries to someone passing by underneath. Mentally ill people, in terms of the old cliché, are mad rather than bad. What is needed is not blame and punishment but some action to treat their illness, that is, to deal with the causes of their bizarre actions so that they will hopefully not act in that way again.

Is determinism the answer, then? Unfortunately, there seem to be serious problems with this argument which suggest the answer 'No'. The first and most obvious is this: if determinism is true, then *no one* is responsible for their actions, whether they are sane or insane. Everyone's actions have causes, which may immediately be thoughts of their own, but must ultimately by something other than thoughts. The sane person who saw Peel's secretary as a harmless employee of an equally harmless politician had no motive for killing him. Putting it rather strangely, the cause of his inaction was this way of perceiving the man. But, if determinism is true, that way of perceiving was itself caused, and its cause was caused in its turn, and so on: if we go far enough back in the chain of causes, we come to something which is not a thought of the person's own, but is something like a brain process, or a process of social conditioning, or something of that kind. So he was not really acting out of free will, and was no more to be praised for *not* killing Peel's secretary than M'Naghten was to be blamed for killing him. Or suppose someone had knowingly assassinated Peel for some more rational reason – perhaps as part of a political *coup d'état.* His action would have its ultimate cause in whatever it was that caused him to belong to this political movement – say, his bitterness at the treatment of his class by Peel's party. Could he help his actions any more than M'Naghten?

This is a difficulty for the argument because it removes all relevant distinctions between crimes committed by the insane and those committed by the sane. It is true that one distinction remains: the causes of insane behaviour are, by definition, different from those of sane behaviour, they are much more unusual. But this creates no *relevant* difference: why should unusual causes be more incompatible with responsibility than usual causes? It would be perfectly possible for a determinist to argue that *no one* is responsible, and that everyone therefore deserves treatment rather than punishment: what the determinist cannot do is mount a special defence on the grounds of insanity. Determinism amounts to adopting Strawson's objective attitude to everyone, sane or insane: to regarding everyone, not as participants in a human relationship with ourselves, but as natural objects, to be handled and managed rather than reasoned with (like the falling slate in the above example).

A second difficulty is this. A scientific approach does not necessarily imply universal causal determinism. To be scientific does indeed mean to seek rational explanations for what happens in the particular field of phenomena that one is studying. But I have argued in an earlier chapter that causal explanation is not the only way in which we can rationally make sense of something, and that in some fields, notably human actions, it is completely inadequate. One could also argue that, even where causal explanation is appropriate, one does not need to go back indefinitely through the chain of causes of causes of causes in order to find the 'real' cause of the phenomenon one is interested in. The slate's falling off the roof is sufficiently explained by the rusting of the nails which hold the slate, combined with the effect of strong winds: in order to explain its fall, we do not need to go further back, to the causes of the rusting or of the sudden rush of wind. The latter are answers to a different question from 'How did the slate come to fall just then?' So, even if our thoughts do have causes, it does not follow that their ultimate cause is not itself a thought of our own: Smith killed Peel because he (Smith) was part of an anarchist plot to overthrow the government; he joined the plot because he was offended at the treatment of the poor by Peel's party. To say that is enough to explain Smith's assassination attempt in a perfectly satisfactory way: we do not need, for example, to inquire for these purposes into whether, say, Smith had anarchist genes or a peculiar neurological structure which attracted him to violence. What matters in explaining his actions is his own thoughts, not what made him the kind of person who might tend to have such thoughts.

More important, however, is the point that not all rational explanation need be causal. If so, then a commitment to science in psychiatry does not imply that we must give a causal or deterministic explanation of mental illness. It has already been conceded that *some* forms of what we regard as mental illness do have causal explanations. Senile dementia, for example, is generally agreed to be caused by deterioration of nerve cells and the formation of plaques in their place. This explanation seems plausible, as already argued, because the mental illness consists in a decline in certain mental *capacities*, and so seems readily explicable by the degeneration of the nervous functioning which makes those capacities possible. In other cases, the argument of earlier chapters has accepted that the *predisposition* to some mental disorders may be causally explained, by for instance unusual brain chemistry. This might apply (whether it does or not is an empirical question which I am not qualified to answer) to at least some cases of depression and schizophrenia: perhaps also to anxiety disorders of various kinds.

If it is possible to give a straightforward causal explanation of a condition as resulting from something which is clearly beyond the sufferer's control, such as deterioration of brain cells through ageing, then that does seem to excuse the sufferer from responsibility for actions which result directly from the condition. It would clearly be wrong, for instance, to blame an Alzheimer's sufferer for failing to recognize her husband of many years, or the doctor who has been treating her for some time. She can't help it. Nor can she really help feeling confused and so fearful because of her situation, and so seeing this strange man not as the doctor who is trying to help her, but as someone potentially bent on attacking her. If so, she is not really to blame for trying to defend herself against his 'attacks', resisting for example his attempts to insert a nasogastric tube by striking him.

The cases where we can give a causal explanation of the predisposition to be in a certain mood or to behave in a certain way are more complex. Suppose, for instance, we can give a biochemical (causal) explanation of the predisposition to depression. This means that we can explain why person A is more likely to react in a depressive way to certain kinds of situation than person B. But person A's actions follow, not from the predisposition, but from the depressive mood. Someone who is in a depressive mood, whether or not they are predisposed to get into such moods, tends to behave in certain ways, such as finding it hard to get up in the morning, and so to hold down a regular job. Whether they are to blame for not turning up to work on time does not therefore depend on whether or not they have a *predisposition* to depression. So the fact of being able to give a causal explanation of that predisposition does not have any bearing on responsibility for actions. The question remains whether and if so why being depressed itself constitutes an excuse. Similarly, whether or not M'Naghten had a causally explicable predisposition to form delusions of persecution does not seem to have any bearing on whether he was or was not to blame for killing Peel's secretary. What we have to ask is why suffering from delusions constitutes an excuse.

My argument in earlier chapters is that, in so far as mental illness consists in distortions of thought, feeling, desire, action and other intentional phenomena, its explanation must be, not causal, but what I have called meaning-explanation. Being depressed is being depressed *about* something. It may be that this 'something' is nothing specific – one may be depressed about 'the world' or 'how things are in general'. But in either case, the explanation of the depression, of what makes this mood one of *depression*, rather than of some other kind – grief or remorse or whatever – must show some relevant way in which the mood or inner feeling is connected with what is outside, its intentional object. That is, it must give the *reasons* for this person to feel depressed in this situation. Similarly, to explain why someone suffers from a delusion, such as the belief that there is a conspiracy by members of the Tory Party against his life, one must give the reasons for holding that belief rather than some other.

Meaning-explanations can be tested empirically, though not in exactly the same way as causal explanations. Some hypotheses about a person's reasons for acting or thinking or feeling in a certain way fit the facts better than others: that is, the more we know about the person and their situation in relevant respects, the more reasonable it becomes to accept one such hypothesis than others. If we knew enough, for instance, about M'Naghten's past life and dealings with the Tory Party, we might well come to see the reasons why he should be suspicious of a conspiracy against him: even though we might not have come to hold such a belief on those grounds. Similarly, if we know that someone feels trapped in a relationship and can see no way out of it, it becomes clear why that person should feel depressed: again, even although we ourselves would not find that relationship oppressive. If meaning-explanations are subject to empirical testing in this way, however, there is nothing unscientific about their use. On the contrary, if they are the only appropriate way to explain human actions, thoughts, feelings and desires, then adopting a truly rational or scientific approach to the study of such human actions etc. *requires* one to seek meaning-explanations rather than, or as well as, causal explanations. The idea that being scientific about psychiatry requires acceptance of universal causal determinism, if that means that human actions must be explained causally, is thus false and confused. We must look elsewhere for a justification of the belief that mental illness is an excuse.

Treatment or punishment?

Meaning-explanations certainly do not seem to be so clearly incompatible with a belief in responsibility in the same way as causal explanations do. Some causal explanations clearly absolve a person from responsibility, by showing that their bodily movements did not in fact amount to an action, for which they could be praised or blamed. For example, if someone with arthritis in the knees stumbles against a glass window and so breaks it, the stumble is probably 'involuntary' in the Aristotelian sense, because it is caused by factors beyond their control, and so is done 'under compulsion'. They are not therefore to blame for breaking the window: their stumble was not an *action* which they performed, but a mere movement of tht body. But actions in the full sense, as I have argued, are to be completely explained by the person's own reasons for performing them: actions are by definition therefore under the person's control, and so cannot be done under compulsion in the way Aristotle describes. If at least some mental illness consists in having thoughts, feelings and desires, or in performing actions, then the question naturally arises, how can mental illness (of this kind) possibly imply diminished responsibility?

Mental disorder has been defined in this book in terms of the degree of unintelligibility of a person's thoughts, feelings, desires and actions. But unintelligibility itself surely cannot constitute an excuse. 'Normal' people may find it hard to understand how Daniel M'Naghten could come to believe that Robert Peel intended to kill him. But equally, those who are not Jehovah's Witnesses may find it hard to understand how someone could come to believe that it was wrong to accept a blood transfusion, even when it would save one's life. It does not follow that an adherent of this faith is not responsible for her refusal of a blood transfusion. In general, human beings are not wholly rational beings, or rather have different views about what is rational, and their choices remain genuine even if their reasons for making them may not be intelligible to those who think differently. Mental disorder, as defined in this book, does not in itself therefore seem to provide grounds for absolving people from responsibility for their actions.

This is of practical importance. It implies that people who commit criminal actions for reasons which most of us find hard to fathom may be called mentally disordered, but may be still as responsible as anyone for their actions. For instance, the mere fact that a paedophile's sexual attraction to small children is something from which most members of society may recoil with horror and incomprehension does not in itself imply that the paedophile is not responsible for his actions. He may plead that he is acting under compulsion, but the unintelligibility of his actions does not, on its own, show this. He certainly does not seem to be acting compulsively in Aristotle's sense, since the source of his actions is not some external force but his own desires. So his behaviour is not, as far as this goes, involuntary in any way which would, in Aristotle's words, 'receive pardon and sometimes pity', rather than 'praise or blame'.

It might be thought that, since we need not only to explain someone's actions in terms of their reasons, but also to explain why they were influenced by *those* reasons rather than any other, we might find here some space for ideas of excusability to enter. Although non-adherents may find the beliefs of Jehovah's Witnesses hard to fathom, they can at least understand up to a point how they might be consistent with other beliefs in a system, and how someone might come to hold such a belief system. Even if we have never experienced it ourselves, we are reasonably familiar with the phenomenon of religious conversion, in which someone comes to accept a new belief system. There are intelligible motives for undergoing such conversion, which even non-believers can appreciate – a desire for identity, a feeling of security from being a member of a group, and, less cynically, an attraction to the moral ideals professed by believers. So we can see why someone might have become a Jehovah's Witness, and, once having done so, have felt obliged to accept that religion's opposition to blood transfusion. In the case of psychotic delusions, or disordered moods, or strange sexual preferences, however, we seem to lack even that degree of ultimate intelligibility. Does that mean that we have, at that level, to seek causal explanations, and might that be the reason why bizarre behaviour or thought becomes excusable?

Unfortunately, that does not seem right. If thoughts and actions have to be explained by the person's reasons, then that leaves no space for causal explanation, however bizarre those reasons are. I am writing this book because I have certain ideas which I want to communicate – that is my reason, in this case a perfectly intelligible one to most people. We can explain why that reason seems important to me, important enough to undertake the labour of writing the book, but that explanation in turn must be in terms of my thoughts. This might not seem to be true. Surely, the explanation of my writing this book must lie in such things as the nature of my professional training and career, the kind of people I associate with and the kinds of things I talk about with them, the direction given to my interests by these discussions, and so on. But in fact it is not these things themselves which have made me want to write this book, but my thoughts about them. I could have had a professional training and career in academic philosophy without ever taking an interest in the philosophy of psychiatry, and so without associating and having discussions with others interested in the same field. No doubt, at some level, none of these interests would have developed at all, still less developed to the point of writing a book about them, if I had not been a certain sort of person – the kind who is inclined to think about certain kinds of problems rather than others, to be persistent about trying to think them through rather than be content with easy answers, and so on. No doubt, too, some part in making me this kind of person was played by such things as my genetic constitution and my early upbringing, neither of which, of course, was under my control. But being the kind of person I am is the product, not of these things alone, but of the way in which I have developed my personality by choices I have made in the course of my experience: I could, for example, with the same genes and early environment have become a psychiatrist rather than a philosopher of psychiatry. And anyway, no matter what the truth of that may be, it is not the kind of person I am by nature which explains my writing of this book, but the interests and reasons which resulted from my nature.

Why should the fact that someone's reasons for doing something are unusual, or even bizarre, in itself make any difference to this situation? Someone may be inclined, genetically and/or as a result of childhood experiences (e.g. of being sexually abused himself), to be sexually attracted to small children rather than, as most of us are, to adults. We may say, if this is so, that he can no more help his feelings than anyone else can help their having sexual feelings about adults. But being a paedophile, in the sense which concerns us, is not merely a matter of having such feelings, but of cultivating them to the point where they become more important than concern for the real welfare of the children concerned, and above all of acting on these desires.

Cultivating feelings in this way and acting on the desires they lead to are both actions, and it is these actions for which one may or may not be held responsible, not for the feelings themselves. Unless one can show some reason why these actions, because of the feelings which inspire them, are in some way beyond the person's own control in a way which is different from actions inspired by sexual feelings for adults, then the mere difference in the feelings will not excuse them. A paedophile, in those circumstances, would be, not mad, but bad.

The problem here could be expressed, in terms used earlier in this book, in this way: is paedophilia a mental *illness* as well as a mental *disorder*? An illness was defined as a disorder from which one suffered because it was not deliberately chosen. In the case of bodily illness, it was not chosen in any sense, because it was explained by causes, natural events outside oneself. Mental illness was argued to be different (except in those few cases like dementia where it could be causally explained). In so far as it involved intentional mental processes and states like thoughts, feelings, and desires, and the actions which they motivated, mental illness required a meaning-explanation. In a sense, therefore, it was chosen, or at least served a purpose for the person in question. But if that choice was made in response to a situation in the person's past which was so problematic that the person could not resolve it with the resources available to him or her at the time, then it could become sedimented into an habitual, and so unconscious, response. This habit could persist, alongside the deliberate or conscious choices of action made in later life, and as such be no longer a matter of deliberate choice: it would be almost *like* something acting on the later person from the outside, even though in a sense it came from the inside. Calling some pattern of thought, feeling or behaviour a mental illness would then be saying that it was not readily intelligible to most people, and furthermore that it could be explained in this special way. And mental illness, in that sense, would make the thought, feeling, or behaviour more excusable: it would not perhaps show that the person absolutely could not help thinking or acting in this way, but it might show that it was not reasonable to expect them to think or act differently.

Whether or not any particular way of thinking, feeling, desiring or behaving counts as a mental illness, and so as an excuse of this kind, is an empirical question, to be answered by trying to find a convincing explanation of this kind. As I have said earlier, as a philosopher I am not professionally qualified to answer such empirical questions: at most, I can say what seems intuitively likely and what fits best with my reading of the evidence collected by those who are qualified. Attempts to answer the question are complicated to some extent by the vagueness of much psychiatric diagnosis. 'Schizophrenia', for example, covers a variety of mental and behavioural abnormalities, some of which may be capable of straightforward causal explanation, but it seems overwhelmingly likely that any of the generally recognized manifestations of schizophrenia which cannot be causally explained can be explained by the special type of meaning-explanation just described. If so, then schizophrenia is definitely an illness, and actions resulting directly from schizophrenia are excusable, in one or other of the ways mentioned. Much the same, it seems, could be said about at least the more severe forms of depression. The case of such disorders as paedophilia is perhaps less obvious. Some paedophiles do indeed seem themselves to have been victims of abuse as children. If their childhood attempts to cope with this experience can be shown to have become sedimented in the form of certain habits of response and behaviour which in later life manifest themselves in paedophilic activities, then perhaps this does imply some diminishment in their responsibility for such activities. As said above, it may not be true even so that they cannot help themselves, but it might be true that it would be unreasonable to expect that they should behave differently. (Another possibility might be that paedophilia might be classified, like autism, as a personality type rather than as a mental disorder, in which case paedophiles would be genuinely incapable of changing their behaviour. This does not seem plausible, but empirical work would be needed to settle the matter).

Does this mean that mentally ill offenders should be treated, rather than punished? Like many of the traditional dichotomies considered in this book, this seems too simple. What do we mean, after all, by the two terms? We punish someone when they have done something wrong, either legally or morally or in some other way. A child who fails an arithmetic test may be punished by getting a bad mark; if the same child tells a lie, they may be punished by being told off by their parents; if an adult parks a car illegally, they may be punished by a fine; if they burgle someone else's house, they may be punished by a prison sentence. And so on. The purposes of punishment are manifold. First, it is a mark of the strength of our disapproval of the action punished: it is a sign to wrong-doers that they have done something which they know to be wrong. The wrong-doer, we say, 'deserves' to be punished, just because she or he has offended: sometimes the metaphor of a debt to society which the wrong-doer repays by undergoing punishment is used. This is why the severity of the punishment is increased as the seriousness of the wrong increases: a murderer, we think, deserves a more severe punishment than someone who steals a sheep. To hold that something is wrong and not to see the point of punishing wrong-doers seems almost logically contradictory, as does seeing that one wrong is greater than another while failing to see that it therefore deserves a greater punishment.

Second, we punish in order to deter other people from doing wrong in the same way – to give them a reason for not acting in the way we disapprove of. Making parking offenders pay a fine is a way of trying to deter people from parking where they shouldn't. Sending burglars to prison is a way of trying to deter burglars. Both of these purposes of punishment are concerned with the well-being of society as a whole, though they depend on the offender accepting the punishment as a just retribution for what they have done. But a third pupose of punishment is at least in part concerned with the well-being of wrong-doers themselves. This is punishment as a means of reforming or rehabilitating the offender. The child who is told off for telling a lie will, we hope, be less likely to tell lies in future; the burglar who goes to prison may be not inclined, as a result, to reoffend in this way. Of course, society as a whole benefits from a reduction in reoffending, but in this case the wrong-doer benefits too.

Punishment serves any of these purposes only if it is in some way unwelcome to the person being punished. Only then will it express social disapproval, or deter, or reform. But it does not follow that it must be harsh or inhuman. Being deprived of one's liberty by being sent to prison, for instance, is unwelcome enough to most human beings: there is nothing in the idea of punishment which implies that prisons must also be places of grinding unpleasantness. Punishment as rehabilitation may indeed require that the environment in which one is punished should be as close as possible to that of normal society: again, the fact that it differs in the essential respect that it is a place of compulsory confinement, separated off from the rest of society, seems to make it as unwelcome as is necessary for it to be called punishment. But punishment as rehabilitation, so conceived, could itself be seen as a form of treatment, aimed at benefiting the person themself by making it possible for the offender to become a part of normal society again. Punishment as expressing the seriousness of the offence, and as deterrent, are distinguishable from treatment, but the line between punishment as rehabilitation and treatment is blurred.

In the case of someone who genuinely and in an absolute sense cannot help doing something which would normally be regarded as wrong, then none of the above functions of punishment have any point. Someone in that position will be unable to recognize the wrongness of what they have done, or therefore the connection between doing it and the punishment which they receive. Equally, someone who cannot help acting in a particular way will clearly not be deterred from so acting by seeing the punishment of others; nor can they be rehabilitated, except in the rather stretched sense that curing them of the condition which makes them unable to help themselves will be a kind of rehabilitation. It is an empirical matter, beyond the scope of this book, to decide who might be in that position, or even if there are any such. But if there are, the only rational and humane response to their offending is the kind of treatment which is distinguishable from anything that could be called punishment. If being responsible means being liable to punishment, then in a very clear sense such people would not be responsible for their actions in the slightest degree.

But there may be other mentally ill offenders (again, it is an empirical matter to say whether there are, and who they might be) of whom it cannot be said that, in the strict sense, they cannot help doing what they do, but of whom it might be said that it was unreasonable to expect them to behave otherwise. These would be people, as was argued above, who, because of their past experiences, have a strong inclination to behave in socially unacceptable ways. It does not seem unreasonable in this case to express the seriousness with which society views what they do, or indeed to try to deter others in a like situation from acting in the same way: in short, punishment in both these senses seems appropriate. They are, in the sense defined above, responsible for what they have done, but they are also particularly appropriate candidates for punishment as rehabilitation, which, as argued, is indistinguishable from treatment, is also fairly obviously appropriate. Given the nature of their condition, the kind of treatment which they require, however, will not be of a kind which is suitable for those who are not responsible for their actions. Rather, it will be one which seeks to enlist their own cooperation – that is, to get them to rehabilitate themselves, by reminding them of the reasons against doing what they have been doing. Programmes to rehabilitate paedophiles by making them face up to the harm which they are doing to children would be a good example: such programmes are both punishment, in that they are unwelcome to the offender, and also treatment in that they are therapy for the condition which gives rise to the offence. We can perhaps say, using rather reluctantly the traditional terms, that those with this kind of mental disorder are *both* mad *and* bad. Once again, the old dichotomies, when they are examined closely, are seen to be far too simple.

Chapter 8

Treatment without consent

The peculiarities of psychiatric ethics

The central claim of this book is that the relationship between psychiatry and general medicine is a tangled one. Simple questions like 'Does the medical model apply to psychiatry or not?' are much *too* simple. In some respects, psychiatry can quite reasonably be regarded as a branch of medicine, but it is not quite like other branches. Mental illness does indeed exist – it is not a myth – but typical mental illnesses are significantly different in character from bodily illness, both in their diagnosis and explanation and consequently in the method of treatment. Some of the methods of treatment appropriate to mental illness are unique, and even those which are similar to the treatments offered in bodily medicine take on a different character from their context. The argument for these claims is essentially that the complex relation between psychiatry and bodily medicine must reflect a proper philosophical under-standing of the relation between the mental and the bodily. Traditional philo-sophical accounts of the mind–body relation, such as dualism and classical materialism, have been rejected, both on philosophical grounds and because they are not adequate for understanding the relation between the treatment of mental and of bodily illness. Dualism represents the mind as a separate domain from the body, governed by special laws of its own: but this fails to explain the similarities and connections between psychiatry and bodily medicine. Classical materialism, on the other hand, treats the difference between mental and bodily illness as one between pathologies of the brain and those of the rest of the body. But this fails to account for the differences between mental and bodily illness. Only Merleau-Ponty's conception of human beings as body-subjects, I have argued, fits the bill both philosophically and clinically.

The complexities in the relationship between psychiatry and bodily medicine are reflected also in psychiatric ethics. Most of the basic principles of medical ethics can be applied to psychiatry, though there are differences in the way in which they may be applied. As Fulford points out (Fulford 1989: xii ff.), ethical concepts seem to enter more obviously into the very heart of psychiatric medicine than they do in bodily medicine. This is in large part because, as Campbell, Gillett and Jones say, the whole nature of the psychiatrist–patient relationship is significantly different from the doctor–patient relationship in bodily medicine (see Campbell, Gillett and Jones 2005: 164 ff.). Because the psychiatrist is dealing with problems affecting the thoughts, feelings, desires and so on of the patient, rather than with the mechanics of the patient's bodily functioning, the clinical relationship necessarily comes closer to an ordinary human relationship between two persons. This is not to deny the importance of the bedside manner in bodily medicine, only to stress the much greater personal involvement which follows from the nature and aims of psychiatry. Psychiatrists can only really help patients with their personal problems if they engage in some kind of dialogue with patients, in which both sides' ideas, values and emotions must play some part. At the same time, however, the relationship can be helpful only if it is genuinely professional, and professionalism precludes too great an involvement on the part of the therapist. There is thus a tension in the psychiatrist–patient relationship, which means 'that the threat to the dignity and self-sovereignty of the patient in psychiatric therapy is much greater than in normal clinical care' (Campbell, Gillett and Jones 2005: 164).

This tension, and the difference between psychiatry and bodily medicine, is most manifest in the case of one particular principle. One of the cornerstones of liberal medical ethics is that doctors must respect the autonomy of their patients. Patients are held to be sovereign, or 'self-determining' (the literal, political, meaning of autonomy), in respect of decisions about their own lives. They alone must therefore, according to this principle, make the final decisions about whether and how they should be treated. Above all, they must have the right to refuse treatment, even when that treatment is clearly medically indicated – that is when, according to the trained opinion of the treating doctor, it is for the patient's own benefit. They must not therefore be hospitalized or treated without their free and genuine consent. This is a liberal principle, in that it subverts the tradition of medical paternalism, in which the doctor was assumed to know best in much the same way that parents are assumed to know better than children what is good for them. The doctor gave the patient orders, based on this superior knowledge, and on the doctor's duty to look after the well-being of patients (the duty of beneficence); it was the patient's duty (and also in the patient's own interests) to obey these orders. Power thus lay on the side of the doctor: the rejection of paternalism restores power to the patient, equalizing the relationship, or rather reversing the power relationship. Doctors may know, because of their training, what is medically good for the patient, but it is assumed that only patients themselves can know what is good *for them*.

All this seems natural in a modern liberal society, in which a central conception is that of the equal human dignity of all citizens. Respect for patient autonomy is an expression of the recognition of the equal human dignity of patients. There is in liberal thought no universal or objective view on, for example, how long life ought to continue or on what 'well'-being consists in. Patients alone, therefore, have the right to accept or refuse treatment, since it is their own life and well-being which is at stake, and therefore their views on how long and in what conditions they wish to go on living have the prior claim to be considered.

But that makes one of the peculiarities of psychiatric ethics even more surprising. So far from seeking to respect the autonomy of psychiatric patients, it is taken for granted that in some cases at least, the wishes of patients about hospitalization and treatment should be ignored and overridden by psychiatrists, and for the patient's own good. The doctors, in other words, are assumed in this case to know better what is good for patients than the patients themselves. Psychiatric patients, again unlike patients with bodily illnesses, may be committed to hospital and treated against their wishes in order to protect others: this raises different ethical issues, which will be considered later in the chapter. These principles are given legal force in most jurisdictions, where there is special mental health legislation stipulating conditions under which patients are to be admitted to hospital or subjected to treatment without their consent and even against their will. The right to refuse treatment, even for life-threatening conditions, which is specifically guaranteed by liberal legislation for those suffering from bodily illness, is thus specifically denied, in some cases at least, to those suffering from mental illness. The very fact that there are such pieces of legislation as Mental Health Acts, but not, for instance, Cardiac Health Acts is an indication that, in the law at least, mental health is not thought of as parallel to the health of the body or any of its parts.

Competence and the right to self-determination

It is worth exploring further why this view is held in the law. The widely accepted argument for refusing or restricting the right to autonomous decision-making in the case of, at least, seriously mentally ill patients is that they are not competent. The right to self-determination is implicitly restricted, in other words, to those who are judged competent. But there are two obvious problems about this. First, if the right to self-determination derives from the duty to respect human dignity, or the worth of the individual, then the restriction of that right to those who are judged competent seems to imply that we have no duty, or only a limited duty, to respect the worth of incompetent individuals. This seems, to say the least, to be a morally dubious position, since it excludes the incompetent from the human community, treating them as less than fully human. Second, it is not clear why even the seriously mentally ill should be judged incompetent to make decisions about their own lives. Who judges them so, and on what criteria?

I shall return to the first problem later, but for the moment let us concentrate on the second. We need to ask first what are the relevant criteria of incompetence in decision-making. A clear and acceptable statement of what most people would understand by 'competence' was given by the US President's Commission for the Study of Ethical Problems in Medicine in 1982:

> Decision-making capacity requires, to greater or lesser degree: (1) possession of a set of values and goals; (2) the ability to communicate and to understand information; and (3) the ability to reason and to deliberate about one's choices.
>
> (President's Commission 1982: 57)

Children, for example, especially small children, would not be judged competent by these criteria, since they have not yet had the time or life-experience to formulate anything which could justifiably be called 'values and goals', and since their abilities both to understand information and to reason about their choices are as yet undeveloped. But even seriously mentally ill adults do not seem to fit the criteria nearly as obviously. An anorexic young woman, for instance, clearly has a goal, that of weight loss; she is intelligent, and seems fully to understand that thereby she is endangering her life; and she has come to the conclusion that achievement of her goal is worth that risk. In what sense, then, we might ask, is she in any different position from, say, an Antarctic explorer who has the goal of reaching the South Pole, recognizes that achieving this goal requires taking serious risks with his life, but nevertheless regards his goal as important enough to him to justify those risks? If the explorer's decision is autonomous and ought to be respected, then why should not the young woman's be treated similarly?

One answer that might be, and has been, given is ultimately derived from the work of the Enlightenment philosopher, Immanuel Kant, who effectively introduced the concept of autonomy as central to moral theory. Beauchamp and Childress, for instance, attribute the authority of the principle of respect for patient autonomy to Kant's argument 'that respect for autonomy flows from the recognition that all persons have unconditional worth, each having the capacity to determine his or her own destiny' (Beauchamp and Childress 1994: 125). The 'unconditional worth' which all persons have, according to

Kant, belongs to them in virtue of their possession of reason: part of what is meant by possessing reason, for Kant, is having the capacity to impose a moral law on themselves, that is, to recognize that something morally ought or ought not to be done just because it is right or wrong in itself, and independently of any interest or desire of their own which may make it appealing or unappealing. For instance, I may recognize that it is right to be honest in my dealings, just because it is, and not because honesty is the best policy – the best way of achieving my own long-term interests.

This recognition, as was said above, is possible for human beings because, and to the extent that, they possess reason. To possess reason, for Kant, is not just to act for reasons (which may include, after all, acting for reasons of self-interest), but to have the capacity to recognize the objective truth of certain moral principles which may conflict with pursuit of our own self-interest. The objectivity of these moral principles consists in their 'universalizability': the fact that they can be shown to be rules which ought to be accepted by any rational being, just as such. In effect, they are the laws which would hold in a society in which all the members were rational, and respected each other as rational beings, and so did not seek to use others as mere means to achieving their own ends. In deciding what it was right to do, we had therefore, according to Kant, to ask whether the maxim or particular principle on which we proposed to act in this case, was such that it could be universalized. That is, could it be phrased as a general law which would apply to all members of such a society equally, and which all could, as rational, autonomous, beings, accept as a principle to act on? This makes it clear what Kant meant by autonomy, and why he thought it played a central role in ethics.

Thus, to have autonomy in the Kantian sense is, as I argued in an earlier article (Matthews 2000: 60 ff.), not so much to have 'the capacity to determine one's own destiny', as to have the power to choose moral principles which will be universal law, applying to all rational beings as such, including oneself. The self who determines actions is, in this way, not myself or yourself, but that abstract rational self which I and you, and all human beings, have in common to the extent that we think and behave rationally. Correspondingly, the destiny which it determines is not mine or yours, but the destiny of rational humanity in general. What we are choosing is not what, in our opinion, is in our own best interests, but what moral principles we shall live by (as potential members of a society governed by reason). In this sense, the explorer who chooses to head for the Pole despite the risks is no more making a rational decision than the anorexic young woman who chooses to starve herself knowing that that means she is likely to die. Either would be acting rationally only if they could will that their maxim could become a universal law. But it is doubtful whether either would really want or (more important) be able to say that incurring the risk of death by acting as they intend to, in pursuit of something which they happen to want to do, is something which every rational being in their situation ought to do. Kant himself would almost certainly say that such a maxim could not be a universal law, and so could not be rational, since it contradicts the fundamental importance of staying alive (cf. Kant 1997: 31 ff.). Nevertheless, there is a difference between them. The Arctic explorer may act irrationally in this case, but he still retains his reason, and so his human worth, in Kantian terms. On the other hand, if mental illness involves a deficiency in reason in the Kantian sense, then mentally ill people are not even capable of exercising autonomy in his sense either, and so are not worthy of respect for their humanity, because that depends on the possession of reason.

It might, of course, be said that Kant's conception of reason and what is rational is anyway much too narrow and abstract to have any point of contact with the realities of human life. We surely include in our concept of rationality much more than the recognition of, and acting upon, universal moral principles: the conscious pursuit of self-interest, for example, even at a cost to others, would generally be regarded as rational, even if deplorable. And we are not so likely nowadays as Kant was to think in terms of universal moral values, which every rational being, just as such, would have to recognize as binding on them. In our more sceptical culture, each person is supposed to work out their own values and preferences: an autonomous being thus becomes someone who does not merely blindly follow the traditional values of his or her society, but lives according to values derived from his or her own personal experience. In this sense, the conscious risk-taker is just as autonomous and rational as the more cautious stay-at-home who prefers staying alive to the excitements of Antarctic exploration. But if so, why is not the anorexic risk-taker also making a rational and autonomous choice which must be respected?

The only difference prima facie seems to be that the explorer's risk-taking seems to be based on a value which he has worked out by personal reflection, and which others may find intelligible, even if they may not share it. It is a reason for doing what he does which he could hope therefore to argue for in debate with others. We think there can be a certain nobility in undergoing hardship and taking risks with one's life, especially if it can be dignified as an essential part of something important like Polar exploration. It may not be something we should call rational, in the sense of prudent, and those who are risk-averse might even call it mad, but it is part of what we might describe as the repertoire of our culture. It is a feature of a liberal culture that it recognizes a greater number of patterns of life as valuable than a more traditional society, thus it is not so clear for us as it was for Kant that only certain laws or values are truly rational.

That range of possible rational values cannot be extended indefinitely: we can come to the end of what even the most tolerant of us can accept as defensible by argument, and so as the outcome of genuinely rational reflection. The anorexic woman's desire to starve herself perhaps does not seem to be intelligible in that way. Her denial of food is not, for instance, a way of making a political or moral point, like that of those who go on hunger strike as part of a protest against what they see as an injustice. Nor is it a way of testing the limits of one's powers of endurance, as it might be, say, in the case of a religious mystic who goes on a fast. We feel that we see the point of refusing food in these other cases: but the point of simply losing weight, to the point where life itself is at risk, or the idea that one is overweight when one clearly is not, simply escapes our comprehension. In the discussion in earlier chapters, it was irrationality in this sense of unintelligibility to normal people which was argued to be the mark of mental disorder.

If that is why we regard the anorexic woman's behaviour as irrational, however, then why should we consider that it affects her autonomy, or her capacity to make decisions? Are we saying simply that her choice of ways to be treated is different from what most of us would make, and so that she ought not to have the right to make a choice? If so, then this seems little more than punishing her for being unconventional: we are treating human worth, membership of the human community, as dependent on social conformity. We can see why anti-psychiatrists like Szasz and Foucault should be led by such considerations to question whether the whole idea of mental illness is a myth, propagated by conventional society in order to keep those who deviate from social convention under control. However, if we do not want to be forced to agree with the anti-psychiatrists, we must find some other and more satisfactory rationale for denying to mentally ill people, as such and in certain circumstances, the right to refuse treatment which is freely accorded to those with bodily illness.

Psychiatric therapy and the restoration of autonomy

I want to propose and then critically examine such an alternative rationale, beginning by returning to the arguments of earlier chapters. The terms 'mental' and 'bodily', I have argued, do not mark out distinct portions of the same domain, like, say, 'cardiac' and 'gastric': they are, rather, ways of referring to different aspects of the life of human beings. Our mental life is our life *as persons*, as beings who relate to the world, and above all to other human beings, in ways which involve meaning, value and purpose – in short, intentional ways. Persons are not immaterial beings, but embodied human beings: we could not, for example, act on the world, or love or hate some other human being, or find some food tastier than others, unless we were embodied creatures. Mental disorder is a disorder in someone's life as a person. But we can also regard our bodies in abstraction from the role which they play in our personal lives, simply as another kind of object in the world, functioning (or failing to function) in accordance with the same laws which govern every other kind of object – the laws of physics and chemistry, and their derivatives in biology. For some purposes, it is useful to treat the body as an object in this way. One of these purposes is that of bodily medicine, which is dedicated to correcting failures of the bodily object to function as we desire it to.

Thus, a bodily illness is one which is taken to affect only our bodies as objects, in this sense: as something considered to that extent apart from ourselves as persons. Seen in this way, our bodies are a kind of possession which we own, like a car or a house. We, as persons, have the sole right to make decisions about what is to happen or to be done with our possessions. In the case of a car, for example, we must decide whether to go on repairing it or to sell it for scrap. In the case of our bodies, we must decide whether we want to go on living, even at the cost of unbearable pain and indignity, or to avoid pain and indignity by being allowed to die. In a liberal, post-Enlightenment culture, as argued above, it is taken for granted that there can be a number of different values to which we can appeal in deciding such questions: each person must decide them for themself, and, since it is the patient's body which is in question, the patient's answer ought to be accepted rather than the doctor's. The political metaphor on which the modern use of autonomy is founded applies here. Sovereign states are autonomous in making arrangements about what is to happen in and to their own territory. It is true that some would argue for the right of humanitarian intervention – the right of other states to invade or use sanctions in order to prevent sovereign states from behaving on their own territory in ways which are regarded as immoral, such as supporting slavery or using torture – but even if we accept the right of humanitarian intervention in international relations, it would not justify medical paternalism. The doctor who ignores a patient's right to refuse treatment is not intervening to prevent the patient from doing something immoral, but to impose on the patient the doctor's own conception of what is 'good for' the patient.

The situation in the case of mental illness, according to the conception which I have argued for in this book, is anyway entirely different. My mind is not one of my possessions, it is me. There may be some point in comparing my relation to the doctor who treats my bodily ills to that towards the garage mechanic who looks after my car, though my body, even for the dualist, is a much more intimate possession than my car. I am the one who formulates ideas about what is desirable in either case. But mental illness, except where it can be identified with brain disease, has been argued to be something other than mechanical problems in one of my possessions: it is a distortion of my being-in-the-world, a change in the very 'me' who formulates ideas about what is or is not desirable in my life. Someone who develops serious clinical depression, for instance, may find their thoughts increasingly turning to suicide, which might well have horrified them in their pre-depressive condition. Or the anorexic young woman mentioned earlier may at one time have been a normal child, with a healthy appetite. Even now, either person may well feel that they both want and do not want what they say they want. The person with depression says (to themself if to no one else) that they want to end it all, but deep down maybe feels they want to stay alive. If they were to be successfully treated for depression, they might well be *glad* that they had not been allowed to end it all. The anorexic woman wants to refuse food, but does not want to die, as she understands full well she will do if she continues to avoid eating. These patients are, in Locke's phrase, 'beside themselves'. They in effect have two selves, so that the question becomes, which of the two should be respected? One self makes decisions with which the therapist can agree, and which could be regarded, reasonably, as the expression of the 'true' self. Is treatment in accordance with its wishes paternalistic, or is it rather properly respectful of autonomy?

Let us explore this further, and try to get clearer about the issues. Talking of there being two selves, and of one as being perhaps more 'real' than the other, is paradoxical. It implies that what someone says, with obvious sincerity, that they want may not be what they *really* want, what they would have chosen if they had done so in full autonomy. We can sometimes make some sense of this idea in cases which do not involve mental illness. For all of us sometimes experience conflicting desires. Someone, say, may want to eat healthily, but may also love chocolate profiteroles. If they are an adult, we could not legitimately simply refuse to let them have chocolate profiteroles on the grounds that *we* thought it was better for them: that would indeed be unacceptable paternalism – treating them like children. But it would be open to us to argue with them, to try and persuade them that it was in their own interests to try to control the less desirable preference. If we succeeded in persuading them, then we should not, paternalistically, be making the decision for them: *they* would have decided for themselves which was the more desirable option. If we did not succeed, then it would indeed be paternalistic to try to prevent them from acting as they chose.

Being a normal (non-mentally ill) adult is being open to the possibility of rational persuasion, but also conversely having the ability rationally to refuse to be persuaded. Both possibilities exist because a normal adult is someone who has formed a hierarchy of preferences: not only do they act on their desires for things, but they desire to act on certain desires rather than others. This account is heavily derivative from Harry G. Frankfurt's distinction between 'first-order desires' – desires to do something or to have something – and 'second-order desires' – desires to have certain desires – which Frankfurt takes as a characteristic of being a person (see Frankfurt 2003).

If we have such a hierarchy of desires, then it seems to make sense of the idea that some of our desires – namely, those which, on reflection, we desire to have – are more truly 'ours' than those which we would prefer not to have. To act autonomously would then be, not to do whatever one (in some sense) wants to do, but to act on those desires which are most truly one's own. In cases of mental illness, however, what seems to happen is that any hierarchical ranking of desires breaks down: the conflicting desires are on the same level, so that there can be no strategy by which individuals can try to control one desire by reminding themselves of their reasons for preferring to act on another. There is thus a sense in which desires become compulsive: the anorexic person cannot help refusing food, the depressive person cannot help feeling suicidal. If so, then there is a lack of autonomy, not because of a lack of reason, but because of a lack of a second-order self which can rank desires in one way rather than another. Mentally ill people are in this sense neither open to rational persuasion, nor able to present a case for continuing as they are which is based on the hierarchy of preferences which they have made their own. They are not autonomous, or self-determining, because in a way they have no self, or no single self, to do the determining.

The job of the psychiatrist is then to help the patient to achieve autonomy by helping them to construct, or to recreate, such a hierarchical ordering, using preferences which they already have. The hope is that, having gained a single self in this way, the anorexic woman will decide that it is better to eat and go on living than to get slimmer and slimmer until one fades away and dies. This, it seems plausible to say, would be the most likely outcome in most cases, but it might, of course, be that the self she formed would be one which placed her desire not to eat over her desire to live: in which case that autonomous decision would have to be respected. In helping her to construct a hierarchy of preferences, however, it may be necessary to disregard one of her presently expressed desires, for instance, her desire not to take nourishment, or her desire to end her life, simply in order that she may live long enough to be able to construct an autonomous self. This, it could be argued, would not be a paternalistic denial of her autonomy, because there is presently no autonomy to deny: rather, it would be respecting her autonomy, in the sense of helping her to develop an autonomous control of her own life. The ethical justification would be like that for emergency life-saving treatment of someone who is unconscious. But it might be suggested that this talk of helping the patient to form her own self as respecting her real autonomy is a piece of verbal trickery, playing around with the notions of real self and autonomy.

In many cases of mental illness, anyway, there is not, or appears not to be, any conflict. The mentally ill person appears at least to have a hierarchy of preferences. It seems at least conceivable, for example, that an anorexic person would *really* sooner die than get fat. Similarly, a depressive person might surely be so convinced of personal worthlessness that they *really* have no desire to go on living. Or, to take a different kind of case, what about those forms of mental illness which crucially involve delusions? Delusive beliefs are by definition not recognized as delusive by the person who holds them. Their consequences therefore are, from the believer's point of view, something to be accepted, just like the consequences of any belief that anyone may hold. Beliefs may make us sad or afraid, for instance: but although sadness and fear are undesirable, if we really believe that the world is this way, then we just have to accept them. There is no real meaning to saying that we have a *desire* to be rid of the beliefs, though we may wish that the world were different, or that we could make it different, from the way we believe it to be. If someone offers us medication which may change our beliefs, we are likely to refuse it, especially if we know from previous experience that this medication has undesirable side-effects. Is a therapist entitled to compel someone to take this medication, just because it seems to the therapist that the patient's belief is deluded? In such cases, to ignore the mentally ill person's expressed wishes does not seem to be a matter of helping them to construct for themselves a form of autonomy out of materials which are already present. It looks more like the psychiatrist's constructing for them a wholly new structure for the self which will conform more to normal conceptions of what is or is not desirable.

The mere fact that the belief in question was false does not seem to provide sufficient grounds in itself for compulsory treatment. Respecting people as individuals is, among other things, respecting their right to believe things which one may regard as false: if their beliefs are to be changed, then that can only legitimately be done by argument, which is not going to work if the belief is delusive, but is often futile also with the deeply held beliefs of normal people. A delusion, however, in the psychiatric sense, is more than a false belief, and indeed, as Fulford points out, in a passage referred to in an earlier chapter (Fulford 1989: 198 ff.) may not be false, and may not be a belief. Even when it is a false belief, what makes it a psychiatric symptom is that it distorts the believer's being-in-the-world – their personal relations to other people and to things, creating problems for the believer in conducting a satisfactory life. Once again, the ethical problem is that the distortion, and the consequent problems, are obvious to the therapist, but not to the patient. Treatment is not comparable to repairing my car, but to creating a new me, one which I have given no sign that I want. Is imposing such treatment without consent or even against the patient's expressed wishes a denial of that patient's autonomy, and so of their worth as a full member of the human community?

Yet a third kind of case is that of those people who have what is generally regarded as a mental disorder, but which might equally well perhaps be regarded as an unusual personality type. Conditions on the autistic spectrum might be seen, as suggested in an earlier chapter, as coming under this heading. If it is true (and this is an empirical matter on which I am not professionally equipped to comment) that autism is the result of innate modes of functioning of the brain, then, although autism is a disorder in the sense of creating problems for those with the condition, it could equally well be described as an identity. Autism is part of what makes someone the person that they are. Ethically speaking, therefore, those with autism have an absolute right to refuse treatment which might make them into a different kind of person. That would be, not the restoration of autonomy (which exists already, as much in autistic as in non-autistic persons), but manipulation of one's personality.

Human dignity

It might be argued that the problem arises from the excessive emphasis in modern liberal medical ethics on the idea of autonomy as the sole criterion of human dignity. Though we may nowadays use a wider sense of rationality than Kant's, we still, like him, treat rationality as the crucial feature of human beings, the source of the worth of humanity. The emphasis on the sovereign rational individual, some feel, portrays the patient as a kind of consumer of health care, making choices between various options which are presented. But this reduces the doctor–patient relationship, it is argued, to a marketplace transaction between sellers and buyers, a cold matter of business in which there is no room for the human relationships of care for vulnerable people which have traditionally formed part of our view of medicine. In the marketplace, psychiatric patients above all lose out, as do the old, the very young and those with serious and debilitating bodily illnesses, none of whom are really in a position to defend their consumer interests, or to engage in rational argument about what is good for them. Far better, the argument goes on, to reinstate medical paternalism, by placing the doctor's duty of beneficence at the head of the principles of medical ethics.

The duty of beneficence is the doctor's obligation to seek first of all the well-being of the patient – surely, it might be felt, the very essence of what is meant by calling medicine a profession, towards which one is called, rather than a trade, which one practises for profit. Is not concern for patients' well-being far more truly a way of showing respect for their human worth than accepting whatever they happen to say they want as the ultimate determinant of treatment? It is saying that their life and well-being are of paramount importance. So on this argument, so far from compulsory treatment of psychiatric patients for their own good showing a lack of respect for their human dignity, it is the clearest possible way of showing such respect.

This argument undoubtedly has considerable appeal to many practising psychiatrists. They are in the profession to help people, and their own conscience impels them to seek what is best for the patient in the long run, while they are aware that the patient is not at present in a position to know what is best. They thus feel understandably impatient with those libertarians who would argue that compulsory treatment, or steps to prevent suicide, are illegitimate interferences in the patient's human rights. Psychiatrists too have rights, they may argue, including the right not to act against one's own conscience. Can we really expect a psychiatrist simply to stand by and allow an anorexic person to starve to death, or a depressive person to commit suicide? Can we even expect psychiatrists to withhold medications which they know would help a schizophrenic patient to stabilize his life, simply because the schizophrenic refuses them?

These arguments certainly have some force, but they also raise problems. There are two interconnected assumptions underlying them. The first is that it is always clear when someone's thoughts, feelings, wishes and so on are pathological, and so should not be taken as representing the patient's 'real' view of the world. The second is that it is clear what is 'for the patient's own good' – to the psychiatrist at least, if not to the patient – but one of the features of modern liberal culture, as said earlier, is that it allows for different and competing conceptions of what is a good way to be. In a more stable, traditional, society, it may have seemed obvious that it was better to stay alive than to die; better to look after oneself and keep oneself clean and tidy than to go around unwashed and unkempt; that certain beliefs were obviously true and others deluded; and that it was better to be in a committed heterosexual relationship than to live on one's own or to be promiscuous. If these things were obvious to any rational being, but not obvious to some individuals, that was a sign that those individuals were irrational, or mad. This also meant that it was in the mad person's own interest, if possible, to restore them to a condition in which these things would seem as obvious to them as to any other normal member of society.

We, however, may not feel so confident that these things are obvious. Perhaps they are not truths of nature but merely expressions of the assumptions of conventional bourgeois society. Even people who are not mad, but are physically ill, may, after all, prefer to be allowed to die rather than suffer certain kinds of intervention, and conventional medical ethics does not regard the withdrawal of treatment in such cases as an abandonment of the duty of beneficence. If the criteria by which we judge people to be mentally ill are nothing more than the standards which hold in conventional society, then the psychiatrist's attempts to return patients to normality, so defined, may equally not be examples of beneficence but of a desire to control others and make them conform to one's own standards. Perhaps the objections of Szasz and Foucault have some force.

We can ask, however, whether these objections are not themselves based on a grossly over-simplified conception of the moral situation. The implication is that there is no valid sense to the idea that certain conceptions of what is good for human beings, what constitutes human welfare, are more rationally based than others. Any propagation of that idea must therefore be simply an attempt by some people to impose their standards on others – whether it is the standards based on their particular religious beliefs, or those holding in some dominant section of society, or whatever. But is that really the only meaning which can be attached to the idea? If we do not think of 'Reason' as a special source of insight into what is good, but simply as the capacity which human beings have to think things out and to argue them out with each other, then we can say that a 'rational' conception of what is good is one which can be defended by argument. A conception which can be defended by argument is one which can be shown to have features which make it appealing to other people than the defender, provided that those others consider it calmly and with an open mind. The defence can of course go on within a single person's mind: individuals can present arguments to themselves in determining what is good, and can contrast that more rational conception of the good with those they may be led to by instinct, or blind emotion, or excessive deference to authority, or wish-fulfilling fantasy.

Rational conceptions of what is good will vary according to context. Someone who is dying of cancer, and aware that she has only a short time to live anyway, may well come to the conclusion that a particular intervention which will somewhat extend her life while diminishing its quality is not worth it. The cost–benefit ratio will be different for her than for someone who knows, or at least thinks, that she has a chance through this treatment of a significant prolongation of life. Each could defend her particular evaluation by arguments which would convince the other that that is what she would conclude *if* she were in the same situation. In a slightly different sort of case, the belief of Jehovah's Witnesses that they should not accept blood transfusions does not immediately appear rationally defensible to those who are not members of that cult, but it becomes more defensible if we take into account the beliefs on which it is based: one can see that, if one shared that starting point, then a rejection of blood transfusions would be a logical conclusion from it. There is not one rationally defensible set of ideas of what is good which will hold for all, despite the differences in their situation, in their belief systems and even, in some cases, differences in their temperament. To this extent, a certain degree of relativism is justifiable.

But some ideas of what is good are not based on argument at all, and cannot be defended by rational argument, even when the context is filled in. Some of the judgements made by people with some serious mental illnesses seem to be like this. They are irrational, not in being the outcome of a lack of reasoning capacity, but in the sense that they are not based on the use of that capacity. In this respect, they are like the irrational prejudices which we all have. If someone feels strongly that computers are a silly modern invention which they have no desire to be involved with, then it is unlikely that they formed that opinion as a result of calm reflection. It is equally unlikely that they could be persuaded to change it by rational argument, or that they could persuade others to share it by presenting arguments for it which would convince someone with an open mind. They would therefore reject any attempt to get them to learn how to use a computer by persuading them that it would improve their life. In the same way, someone with anorexia who believes it would be better to die thin than to live fat has not formed that view by careful reflection. Whatever has caused her illness has also made her more inclined to jump to this conclusion than to reflect calmly about the matter. And while she remains in this condition, she will be unshakable by the arguments of others and may well reject the idea that she is in a condition which needs help.

The idea that she needs help, and that her illness-based view of the world is irrational and damaging to her own best interests, may not, however, be just an alternative view or just a view based on equally irrational bourgeois prejudices. It is one which looks as if it could be defended by arguments which anyone considering them calmly could accept. Losing weight cannot be an end in itself, but only a means to an end: it may be a means to make one look more attractive to others, or, more importantly, to improve one's health. In either case, there is a limit beyond which losing weight does not need to go, and must not be allowed to go, and that limit comes well before the point of starvation. A dead person can not be attractive to others, and, even more obviously, can not be healthy. The very fact that these arguments are boringly obvious shows that they offer a rational objection to the anorexic's judgement. The only thing which is preventing the anorexic herself from accepting these arguments is her illness: if she were successfully treated for her illness, then we can predict with some certainty, based on similar cases in the past, that she would accept them and change her judgement. Even though she may now refuse the necessary treatment, therefore, it would still be an act of beneficence on the part of a psychiatrist to impose that treatment on her against her wishes – an act for which she herself might well thank the therapist.

Would it however show a lack of respect for her autonomy? Would it, as it was earlier expressed, be more like creating a new identity for her? To answer 'No' to these questions is to hold that successful treatment for mental illness is not the construction of a new person, but the release of the person's own self from the illness which was distorting it. That in turn implies that one's own self is the one which forms its values, its ideas of what is good, through reasoning and reflection. It would, of course, be utterly unrealistic to imagine that 'forming through reason and reflection' meant 'forming as a result of conscious deliberation'. Very few people, if any, are as reflective as that, but there could still be a sense in which, in the course of normal development, we arrive at various ideas about what is good, on the basis of human instinct, but also on that of personal experience, discussion with others, reading, and so on, which could be defended if need be by the kind of rational argument which has been mentioned. These ideas of what is good are likely to vary to some extent from one cultural setting to another, but they are not simply the conventional ideas of our cultural setting – indeed, they are often formed through rebellion against such conventions. Mental illness distorts these ideas, either through preventing normal development and so the growth of a coherent rationally defensible view of things; or through disrupting an already formed view of things, making it less coherent and less rationally defensible. But it does not necessarily remove the possibility of rational argument, and beneficence itself requires, if this is so, that the psychiatrist makes every effort to persuade the patient to accept the clinically indicated treatment: beneficence in that case includes respect for autonomy. If rational persuasion seems impossible, however, then beneficence seems to trump respect for autonomy, precisely in the name of respecting the patient's humanity.

Acting out of beneficence in treating psychiatric patients against their wishes is thus not necessarily failing to respect their human dignity in any important sense. The psychiatrist acts, not to impose their own values on patients, but out of a prediction of what patients themselves will afterwards acknowledge to have been what they really wanted all along. There are undoubtedly dangers in this recommendation. Above all, such predictions are notoriously unreliable. It is only too easy for psychiatrists to think that what they think would be best for patients is what patients themselves will be bound to accept as best for them, once they can think rationally again. Psychiatrists are human beings too, and their picture of what mental health consists in is as likely as anyone else's to be derived from their own cultural background. The aim has to be, not to direct the patient to any particular conception of what is good, but to enable them once more (or perhaps for the first time) to form conceptions of the good by rational reflection of the kind described. Mental health is having the same degree of control over how one conducts one's life as most of us have, not being conformist to the standards of respectable society. But it is only too tempting to believe that a conception of the good is only a *rational* one, and so genuinely autonomous, if it happens to coincide with one's own. There is always a danger, therefore, that, although the declared aim of psychiatric treatment in such cases may be to restore rational control of one's life, what is in fact aimed at is the imposition of conventional middle-class standards.

That this danger exists is undeniable, but perhaps it simply has to be accepted, since there seems no viable alternative: to accede to patients' expressed wishes to harm or neglect themselves is simply a dereliction of the duty to care for patients' real welfare. Awareness of the risks can at least make psychiatrists more ready to take steps to avoid or minimize them. It is interesting and significant, too, that most mental health legislation builds in safeguards restricting the right to treat without consent. For example, there are requirements for more than one person to make such decisions, and for regular review of decisions which have been made, and there are restrictions on the use of very radical interventions such as psychosurgery, which may, by affecting brain function, undermine a patient's ability to reflect and to form an integrated conception of themselves. In an imperfect world, minimization, rather than complete eradication, of risk, and the possibility of retrieving situations which have gone wrong, may be the most we can hope to achieve.

Harm to others

As was mentioned above, mental health legislation usually includes provision for compulsory admission to hospital and treatment, not only for the patient's own good but in order to prevent harm to others. This raises different sorts of ethical issues from those which have been discussed in the earlier part of this chapter: preventive detention of this sort could not be described as a form of medical paternalism. It is motivated, not by the doctor's duty of beneficence towards the patient, but by the fear of the consequences for society at large if the patient is not put out of harm's way. It does, however, raise questions of the patient's human rights, of the ability of people to live their lives freely and in that sense autonomously. No one, of course, has the right to do harm to others, and so it is not contrary to anyone's rights to imprison them if they have been found guilty, after due process of law, of having committed some harm. The ethical problem arises when people are, in effect, detained because they are thought likely to commit harm *in the future*, or when they are considered to be harmful in ways which do not fall under the law and which are not subject to proper legal trial.

Do we (that is, society at large) have the right to detain people who have not, as yet, committed any crime, and have certainly not been found guilty of a crime in a properly constituted court of law, simply on the grounds that they *might* commit a crime in the future? In most cases, the answer of the majority of people in a modern society would be 'No', but in the case of people with mental illness, the right to detain people in this way (subject, of course, to certain safeguards) is enshrined in law. How can we explain this, if any rational explanation is possible at all? One possible answer would be that it is an important difference between people with certain kinds of mental illness and those who are not mentally ill, that it is much easier to predict that they may behave violently to others. Furthermore, the violence they are likely to commit is often of a worse kind. Finally, it is likely to be inflicted randomly and so to affect those who have no connection with the perpetrator, and so least expect to be attacked in this way. But, first, the facts do not appear to support this argument. Psychotics are not always inclined to violence, anyway, and the predictions of violent behaviour by mentally ill people, judged by the outcomes, are varyingly reliable. It is far from clear that predictions about mentally ill people are any more likely to be accurate than those about people with no diagnosed mental disorder. Certainly, those who are released from detention, either in a prison or in a mental hospital, back into the community on the basis of predictions that they will not re-offend quite often falsify these predictions, much to the dismay and anger of the general public. It seems quite likely therefore that some of those confined in hospital on this basis would never have offended in the predicted way. These people would be confined although they were, to coin a phrase, 'doubly innocent' – neither having committed an offence nor likely to do so in the future – and that seems plainly unjust.

Suppose future advances in psychology, or perhaps in genetics, were to make it possible to predict violent behaviour with absolute certainty. (This seems to be an almost meaningless supposition, but it will serve the purpose of examining the issue in more depth.) Or suppose someone is openly and explicitly threatening to do harm to someone. A psychiatrist would be able then to say 'Patient X will certainly do some harm to someone unless he or she is detained in a secure place.' Would this be morally acceptable? This would depend on how far it is morally permissible to go in order to prevent future harm to someone else. If the harm to be prevented is both certainly predictable and great (X would murder someone, for instance), then it might outbalance the harm done to X by confining them in a place where they would be humanely treated, and where they would be spared the guilt and shame of committing harm to another innocent person. The rights of the potential victim not to be harmed in this way surely trump the rights of X to be allowed to go about freely. The balance would obviously change, however, as the degree of harm to the victim diminished and/or the probability of the harm being done decreased. If X was simply a bit of a nuisance to his neighbours, then that would not entitle anyone to have him detained, unless it were paternalistically, for his own good.

What about treatment while he was detained? If the treatment could be justified for his own good, then we are back with the arguments about paternalism. But suppose the primary aim of the treatment was to reduce the chance of X's re-offending. He might, for example, be given a sedative in order to make him less inclined to violence. Or, much more radically, he might be chemically castrated to make him less able to commit sexual offences. The good to be achieved by treatments of these kinds would be to protect others from serious harm, but it is, to say the least, highly questionable in these cases whether the balance between the rights of others and the rights of X himself would have been struck. The harm done to X would be that of treating him like a thing, not a human being. People's bad behaviour can be legitimately changed only by persuasion to see that what they have been doing or proposing to do is unacceptable. But in this case, X's behaviour would have been manipulated, so that what he did in future would not have been the result of his own choice. He would have been reduced to the level of a robot. Even if X *chose* to undergo this treatment, that would not necessarily make it morally tolerable. To choose to be dehumanized is choosing to be in a state where one can make no more choices, where one's existence is determined not by one's own will but by the requirements of others, and that does not seem like a morally legitimate choice to make. A sex offender or someone prone to outbursts of anger can legitimately seek help in learning to control his own impulses, but not treatment designed to remove those impulses altogether: the former is compatible with his continuing humanity, the latter is not.

Thus, in law and ethics as well as in modes of therapy and their intellectual foundations, mental disorders are both different from and in some ways similar to bodily diseases, at least as traditionally conceived. That they do is both a consequence and a confirmation of the account of the relationships of mental and bodily life, respectively, to us as persons which is contained in Merleau-Ponty's conception of human beings as body-subjects. The most important conclusion of all to derive from the arguments of this book, however, is that it is just as dangerous to indulge in simple dichotomous thinking about the ethics and law of psychiatry, as about the clinical explanation and treatment of those conditions we have come to call mental disorders.

References

American Psychiatric Association (1994) *Diagnostic and Statistical Manual of Mental Disorders*, Fourth Edition. Washington DC: American Psychiatric Association.

Aristotle (2004) *The Nicomachean Ethics*.Translated by J. A. K. Thomson, revised with notes and appendices by Hugh Tredennick, Introduction and Further Reading by Jonathan Barnes. London: Penguin Books.

Beauchamp T. L. and Childress J. F. (1994) *Principles of Biomedical Ethics*, Fourth Edition. New York/Oxford: Oxford University Press.

Bolton D. and Hill J. (2003) *Mind, Meaning and Mental Disorder, The Nature of Causal Explanation in Psychology and Psychiatry*, Second Edition. Oxford/New York: Oxford University Press.

Boorse C. (1989) 'On the distinction between disease and illness'. Reprinted in T. L. Beauchamp and LeRoy Walters (eds) *Contemporary Issues in Bioethics*, Third Edition, pp. 90–96. Belmont, CA: Wadsworth Publishing Co. (Originally in *Philosophy and Public Affairs*, 1975, **5, 1**, 49–68).

Campbell A., Gillett G. and Jones G. (2005) *Medical Ethics*, Fourth Edition. Melbourne/Oxford/New York: Oxford University Press.

Churchland P. M. (1981) 'Eliminative materialism and the propositional attitudes', *Journal of Philosophy*, **78**.

Descartes R. (1985) 'Discourse on the method'. In J. Cottingham, R. Stoothoff and D. Murdoch (translators), *The Philosophical Writings of Descartes*, Vol. I. Cambridge/New York: Cambridge University Press.

Foucault M. (1989) *Madness and Civilization: A history of insanity in the age of reason*, translated by Richard Howard. London: Routledge.

Frankfurt H. G. (2003) 'Freedom of the will and the concept of a person'. Reprinted in G. Watson (ed.), *Free Will*, Second Edition, pp. 322–36. Oxford/New York: Oxford University Press. (Originally published in *Journal of Philosophy*, 1971, **68**, 5–20).

Fulford K. W. M. (1989) *Moral Theory and Medical Practice*. Cambridge/New York: Cambridge University Press.

Heidegger M. (1962) *Being and Time*, translated by J. Macquarrie and E.Robinson. Oxford: Basil Blackwell.

Husserl E. (1960) *Cartesian Meditations*, translated by D. Cairns. The Hague: Martinus Nijhoff.

Husserl E. (1970) *The Crisis of European Sciences and Transcendental Phenomenology: An Introduction to Phenomenological Philosophy*. Translated by D. Carr. Evanston, IL: Northwestern University Press.

Jaspers K. (1997) *General Psychopathology*, 2 vols, translated by J. Hoenig and M. W. Hamilton. Baltimore, MD: The Johns Hopkins University Press.

Kant I. (1997) *Groundwork of the Metaphysics of Morals*, translated by M. Gregor. Cambridge/New York: Cambridge University Press.

Kendell R. E. (1975) 'The concept of disease and its implications for psychiatry', *British Journal of Psychiatry*, **127**, 305–15.

Kenny A. J. P. (1969) 'Mental health in Plato's Republic', *Proceedings of the British Academy*, **5**, 229–53.

Laing R. D. (1965) *The Divided Self*. London: Penguin Books.

Locke J. (1975) *An Essay concerning Human Understanding*, ed. P. H. Nidditch. Oxford: Clarendon Press.

Matthews E. (1995) 'Moralist or therapist? Foucault and the critique of psychiatry', *PPPL: Philosophy, Psychiatry, and Psychology*, **2**(1): 19–30.

Matthews E. (2000) 'Autonomy and the psychiatric patient', *Journal of Applied Philosophy*, **17**(1): 59–70.

Matthews E. (2002) *The Philosophy of Merleau-Ponty*, Chesham, Bucks: Acumen Publishing Ltd.

Matthews E. (2003) 'How can a mind be sick?'. In B. Fulford, K. Morris, J. Sadler and G. Stanghellini (eds) *Nature and Narrative: an introduction to the new philosophy of psychiatry*, pp.75–92. Oxford/New York: Oxford University Press.

Matthews E. (2004) 'Merleau-Ponty's body-subject and psychiatry', *International Review of Psychiatry*, **16**(3): 190–8.

Matthews E. (2005a) *Mind: Key Concepts in Philosophy*. London/New York: Continuum.

Matthews E. (2005b) 'Laing and Merleau-Ponty'. In S. Raschid (ed.) *R. D. Laing: Contemporary Perspectives*, pp. 80–98. London: Free Association Books.

Matthews E. (2006) *Merleau-Ponty: A Guide for the Perplexed*. London/New York: Continuum.

Matthews E. (forthcoming) 'Suspicions of schizophrenia'. In M. Chung and G. Graham (eds), *Reconceiving Schizophrenia*.Oxford/New York: Oxford University Press.

Merleau-Ponty M. (2002) *Phenomenology of Perception*, translated by Colin Smith, (Routledge Classics edition), London/New York, Routledge.

Merleau-Ponty M. (2004) *The World of Perception*, translated by Oliver Davis. London/ New York: Routledge.

Moore M. S. (1984) *Law and Psychiatry: Rethinking the relationship*, Cambridge/New York: Cambridge University Press.

Moran D. and Mooney T. (eds) (2002) *The Phenomenology Reader*. London/New York: Routledge.

Place U. T. (1956) 'Is consciousness a brain-process?', *British Journal of Psychology*, **47**, 42–51.

Porter R. (2002) *Madness: A Brief History*. Oxford/New York: Oxford University Press.

Ryle G. (1949) *The Concept of Mind*. London: Hutchinson's University Library.

Sadler J. Z., Wiggins O. P. and Schwartz M. A. (eds) (1994) *Philosophical Perspectives on Psychiatric Diagnostic Classification*. Baltimore, MD/London: Johns Hopkins University Press.

Smart J. J. C. (1959) 'Sensations and brain-processes', *Philosophical Review*, **68**, 141–56.

Strawson P. (2003) 'Freedom and resentment'. Reprinted in G. Watson (ed.) *Free Will*, Second Edition, pp. 72–93. Oxford/New York: Oxford University Press. (Originally published in *Proceedings of the British Academy*, 1962, **48,** 1–25).

Szasz T. (1972) *The Myth of Mental Illness: Foundations of a Theory of Personal Conduct.* St Alban's, Herts: Granada Publishing Ltd.

The President's Commission for the Study of Ethical Problems in Medicine and Biomedical and Behavioral Research (1982) *Making Health Care Decisions: The Ethical and Legal Implications of Informed Consent in the Patient-Practitioner Relationship*, report, vol. 1. Washington, DC: US Government Printing Office.

Williams B. (1978) *Descartes: the Project of Pure Enquiry*. London: Penguin Books.

Wittgenstein L. (1953) *Philosophical Investigations*, translated by G. E. M. Anscombe. Oxford: Basil Blackwell.

World Health Organization (1992) *The ICD-10 Classification of Mental and Behavioural Disorders: Clinical descriptions and diagnostic guidelines*. Geneva: World Health Organization.

Index